My best

Joan Schreiner

# STILL HERE!

# STILL HERE!

*Taking Charge of
Your Health Care*

Joan Schreiner

**To order additional copies of this book, contact:**
Xlibris Corporation
1-888-795-4274
www.Xlibris.com
Orders@Xlibris.com
22261

# CONTENTS

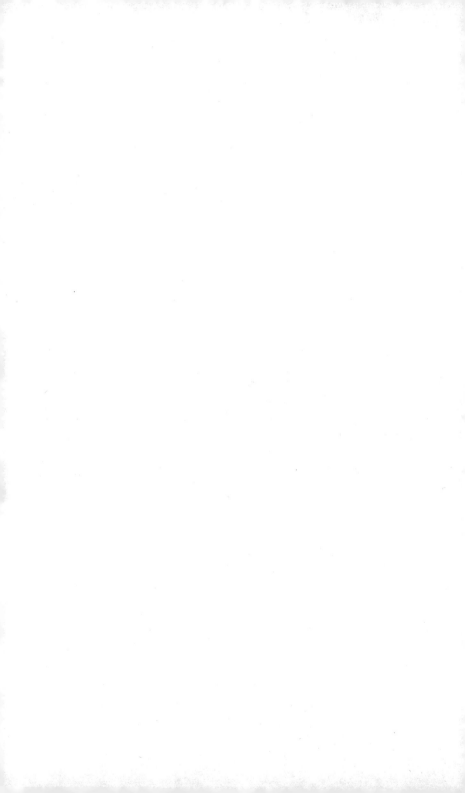

This book is dedicated to my husband, David Nagel.
He simply refused to let me give up.

# Acknowledgements

So many people have helped along the way that it is impossible to name them all here. However, I would like to acknowledge those who have provided almost continual support over the last ten years. Their many acts of kindness are beyond counting.

My gratitude belongs to my parents, Bob and Dorothea Schreiner, my brother Tim and sister Lynn. Many, many thanks to my good friends and unfailing supporters: Joyce Farrell and Brian Wandell, Joanne Tyler, Beau and Kathleen Watson, Anita Schiller, Lucy Shapiro, Nina Katz and Craig Upson, Emmett Donahue and Sandy Hart.

For all of her talents in ministering to the community, my deep appreciation to Elaine Dornig of Bay Area Breast Cancer Network.

My medical heroes include oncologists Dr. Alex Tseng of SouthBay Oncology and Dr. Debu Tripathy, formerly of UCSF and now at the University of Texas Southwestern; breast surgeon Dr. Jocelyn Dunn; mammographer/radiologist Dr. Diana Guthaner; neurologist Dr. Steven Chang of Stanford; and Dr. Stanley Rogers of UCSF, pioneer of the radio-frequency ablation procedure.

Although a late participant in this journey, I am grateful to Margot Wolf, who became a friend first, and then lent her considerable editing expertise to help this book become even better.

Thanks to my stepdaughter, Rebecca, who not only lent her support but also contributed her expertise at graphics in designing the cover for this book.

A very special thanks to ALL of the nursing staff at SouthBay Oncology. You are simply the best.

And to my husband, David, my editor-in-chief. His encouragement and many contributions to this book have been of enormous value.

# Preface

This book was borne from my ongoing battle with breast cancer, now in its tenth year. Along the way, I have learned much about breast cancer in particular, and the front lines of cancer research in general. My personal story has been complex, constantly changing, and fraught with all of the emotional ups and downs of dealing with a chronic, life-threatening illness. I have survived multiple chemotherapy rounds, breast surgery, reconstructive surgery, a stem cell transplant, spinal cord and brain radiation, CyberKnife radiosurgery, radio-frequency ablation to my liver and, most recently, brain surgery. I am constantly reading about new therapies, attending research symposia, and conferring with experts across the country. I have tried almost every traditional therapy as well as a host of new treatments available only within the past couple of years. The result is that I have become not only an expert on breast cancer but skilled at dealing with the medical establishment.

These skills developed over time as I was confronted with new and unique situations concerning both my health and our health care system. Prior to breast cancer, my life as a patient had been limited to check-ups and routine x-rays. Like most people, I squeezed in medical appointments only when absolutely necessary, usually juggling them with the demands of work (work usually receiving top priority), and never expected that a serious medical problem could occur when I was only in my thirties. There was no precedence for this in my family, and I thought I had done all the "right" things—exercised regularly, ate plenty of fruits and vegetables, got enough sleep, and kept the weight off. Even when I was confronted with symptoms, my husband had to urge me to make a doctor's appointment.

I started off as most people do, believing that if I went to the well-known medical facility I had been visiting since childhood and followed their instructions exactly, I would be healed by a sympathetic, "Marcus Welby-like" physician. I expected this doctor to be totally competent, have my best interests at heart at all times, be up to date on all of the latest treatments, and to look into the future for those not even available yet. My expectations gradually began to fall by the wayside as I came to realize the high cost I would pay if mistakes were made. With an initial misdiagnosis and consequent six-month delay in treatment, this awakening was shocking. Nevertheless, it *still* took me some time to develop the base of knowledge and skills I have needed to fight the ongoing battle.

The issues and decisions most patients are faced with are generic to all forms of serious illness. Due to my involvement in the breast cancer community, I am regularly called upon to talk to newly diagnosed women. Although many of them want to know about treatment options, I find that I actually spend more time providing a set of tools with which to deal with the path that lies ahead, strongly encouraging them to *take charge of their medical care from the very beginning.* It is a long and arduous path, with critical decisions to be made at regular junctions. To make the best possible choices, one must develop problem-solving skills, a base of knowledge about the illness, and a network of resources and support. I often spend a couple of hours on the phone with people who are referred to me through mutual friends, usually feeling the need to leave them with something more concrete that they can digest at their own pace.

In developing this guide, I have drawn heavily upon my experiences and, although the book inevitably focuses on breast cancer, I believe that many of the principles apply to almost any serious illness, and most certainly to other forms of cancer. Where appropriate, I share specific resources for breast cancer, but similar sources are available for other types of cancer.

My book starts with some reflections on my own story and the therapies I have undergone so far. As I celebrate my tenth year of survival, I look back on the many treatments as well as the strategies that I developed along the way. While the initial chapter covers "what happened," the rest of the book details how I did it. The timeline is the same for anyone with a serious illness: diagnosis, followed by the search for a doctor and/or medical team, and an initial decision-making process. Patients must learn about the medical system infrastructure as well as how the care they receive is influenced by medical hierarchy and the insurance industry. Issues concerning maintenance of health insurance are covered in a separate chapter.

For patients facing an ongoing condition, I offer a chapter covering resources that go well beyond basic information. Following this is a final argument as to why the *Take Charge* patient is the model of the future. I conclude with coping strategies, including advice to friends and family on how they can help. I have provided a list of summary points for each topic whenever possible.

It is my sincere hope that anyone reading this book will find this to be a useful approach and resource. I know that everyone has their own way of dealing with illness, and that my way may be a bit too analytical for some. While I do not address non-traditional or religious approaches, I appreciate their intrinsic value. In fact, there are many techniques that can complement traditional medicine.

I am also aware that an aggressive approach to managing your own health care may seem daunting to some. However, based on my own experience, it is not as difficult as it appears, and I believe that you will *increase your survival* by managing the situation assertively. You can even survive when mistakes are made along the way.

Although I have continued to have an active professional life throughout my illness, staying alive has been my primary job and goal. This focus on *survival* caused the paradigm shift to taking charge. It required me to become more assertive with people I didn't know well, and less concerned about whether I behaved like a "nice" patient. While I don't think I alienated too many people, I certainly had significant conflicts with some and learned to accept this as part of the process. The fact is, I am "still here" and have managed to maintain a reasonably good quality of life. I am convinced that the strategies I have used and the ability I have developed to *take charge* have been absolutely essential to my survival.

As I began to write and necessarily had to re-live painfully everything that had happened to me, I thought, "My god! How did I survive all this?" This book is designed to teach you—or someone you care about—how to do it, too.

# Chapter 1

## My Story: Reflections on a Personal Journey

I awoke from the biopsy suffering from chills, not yet fully awake, and with the surgeon peering in my face. Despite his optimism going into the surgery, which he said I could "schedule at my convenience," he now rapidly communicated that it "didn't look good." He had found "multiple lesions," and he would let me know in a few days. With that, he disappeared, and my husband and I were left to digest this information. This was our introduction to cancer and the medical system. It also foreshadowed many things to come.

Among the most fearsome three words in English are, "You have cancer." When I first heard these words over the phone just a few days later, my reaction was shock, disbelief, anger and, eventually, adjustment to the reality of the situation. As many patients with a serious illness will attest, it had a profound impact on my personality and outlook on life. Not surprisingly, life became quite *alive* for me—precious. At the same time, it became much more chaotic, unpredictable, and uncontrollable. I simultaneously became more determined and more humble, angrier but also more grateful to simply be here. Living on the edge had given everything both new contradictions and new meaning.

I became much more relaxed and, although still ambitious in my career, I was less concerned about day-to-day irritations. I even had a calming affect on my colleagues. I often found myself saying that there was no need to worry, that the immediate problem was "not life-threatening" and we would work it out. I joked with one of my managers that I was no longer bothered by having to deal with rush-hour traffic. On a more important personal level, I lost any remaining shyness I had suffered from as a young woman and began immediately to reach out and build a strong medical network. This ability, born out of necessity, had a positive impact not only on my medical life but also, later on, professionally.

The whirlwind of those first several weeks was enormously stressful, yet in an unexpected way, I was able to draw upon all of my life experiences. Ironically, I had completed my undergraduate major in the natural/biological sciences and worked briefly as a chemist before going to graduate school for an MBA. An early interest in medicine, coupled with business skills developed during the course of my professional career, proved to be helpful in getting started in my new "job". A natural stoicism came to my rescue many times, allowing me to remain calm in the face of impending disaster.

While I immersed myself in the short term decision process, I was also forced to deal with the reactions of my friends and colleagues. I was warned by my new cancer network friends that I would find this development surprising, even incomprehensible, and I did. On the positive side, many people, including some whom I had only considered acquaintances, did offer support and friendship. I was dumbfounded to hear personal confessions from some concerning difficulties in their own lives of which I was unaware. One friend confessed that she had been dealing with depression for quite some time. Another announced that she had been seeing a therapist. I soon learned that the receptionist in my building had been treated for brain cancer when she was just a child and she began greeting me warmly when I arrived each morning. Another administrator, who was fighting lymphoma, immediately called to offer her support. In retrospect, I think this was their way of empathizing with my plight, but I was unprepared for their revelations.

On the negative and more disturbing side, I also found several people who ran as quickly as they could in the opposite direction. As bad as this was at work, it was much more upsetting when they were personal friends. One friend with whom I'd been close and known for nearly twenty years suddenly disappeared during the first year of my treatment. Although I have resumed contact since then, the friendship has never really recovered. My colleagues' behavior in the office was much more subtle. I noticed that a few reduced communication with me—or avoided it altogether—occasionally even going out of their way so they wouldn't have to make any direct physical contact. In meetings, some wouldn't or couldn't look me in the eye, but I could see their distress at my changed appearance.

The first surgical procedure required a brief hospitalization followed by many weeks of physical therapy. The recovery process forced me to take about a month off from my job as a division controller at Silicon Graphics, but I insisted on returning on a part-time basis during my seven months of chemotherapy. At the time, this was an emotionally important decision for me, as I felt that staying home was tantamount to "giving in" to the illness. My employers' initial reaction had been supportive, and they almost immediately offered to keep the entire thing "quiet" and to fill in for me whenever I was unable to perform. I rejected this since I had always prided myself on my performance: the last thing I wanted was to be viewed as someone who couldn't deliver for reasons unknown. I insisted on a full and immediate disclosure to everyone. This is, of course, a matter of personal choice and many people choose to keep their condition strictly private. There are good reasons for this, including the possibility of job discrimination, which is often vague and difficult to prove.

In retrospect, I have to admit that going back to work so quickly was difficult for me as well as disruptive for my colleagues who had to deal with a co-worker who was obviously suffering from the effects of chemotherapy. The hair loss was the most challenging consequence. At first, I embraced the notion that I would not be embarrassed by this, alternating between a shoulder-length brown wig (I had worn my hair short) and an ever-changing set of hats and scarves. In reality, I was devastated and clung to the hope that the daily shedding would end. This was a mistake, and during subsequent chemotherapies, I allowed my husband, Dave, to shave my head the minute my hair started feeling loose. I now advise all new patients to do this, since it gets the process over quickly instead of perpetuating the daily trauma. There are many good wig stylists and a high-quality wig made from human hair is almost undetectable.

I was also challenged with several hospital stays, due to the impact of the chemo on my immune system. On one occasion, I continued to lead a group through a budgeting meeting even as I felt my temperature steadily increasing. When I finally packed up and decided to drop by my physician's office, I had a 102° fever and a white blood count which was so low as to be almost immeasurable. Alarmed, the doctor not only immediately admitted me to the hospital, he even drove me there in his own car!

Then there was the reconstruction following my breast surgery, which is considered "optional" by the medical community, but necessary by many patients. The two common techniques are the transplantation of tissue from elsewhere on the body (known as a "tram flap"), or the use of a saline implant. I opted for the implant, which required the use of a tissue expander, a device which is surgically implanted and then slowly filled with saline ("expanded") during the course of several office visits. Over several months, the pressure from the saline serves to stretch the skin (much as pregnancy does), which then allows for the insertion of the final implant.

My first attempt at the final implant involved making a plaster cast of my remaining "good" breast on the right side. I was amused as the technician proceeded to layer me with plaster. I could not help but laugh and just had to ask, "Now, what exactly do you tell people you do for a living at cocktail parties?"

The final implant, unfortunately, did not look as good as I had expected, and I insisted we try again. After three attempts, the size and symmetry finally met my expectations. I looked and felt much better after this.

Over the course of about nine months, the therapy was completed and my life returned to normal. My reaction to having survived was to throw myself into a number of volunteer projects related to breast cancer, including becoming a very early adopter of the internet in 1994, and implementing one of the first public-access internet facilities for women's health care at an organization in Palo Alto. As a result, I briefly found myself at the intersection of cancer and the internet and was interviewed extensively by cancer periodicals, local newspapers, and even the *Wall Street Journal* (my proverbial fifteen minutes of fame). I also organized and produced two comprehensive medical conferences on breast cancer on-site at Silicon Graphics (my employer at the time), spoke at other local medical conferences, and even served as a reviewer on a panel for BCRP grants (BCRP, which stands for Breast Cancer Research Program, is a taxpayer funded granting entity in the state of California. ) While I believe this was helpful to the community at large, it was also clearly helping me.

Every cancer patient harbors the fear, whether he or she says so or not, that the illness will return. This diminishes as time goes by, as most recurrences happen within the first four to five years. At the end of my fourth year out, I remember breathing a big sigh of relief as my doctor and I congratulated each other. I thought I could put the experience behind me at that point and made a decision to leave big company life and try my hand at a start-up (Silicon Valley's term for a newly formed technology company). As a precaution, I went in for a check-up and my doctor gave me a clean bill of health.

I was invigorated by the challenges and diversity of life in a small company. Only four months into the job, however, another check-up revealed a heightened set of tumor markers. A follow-up chest scan confirmed our worst fears: a massive recurrence in my lungs. Although I had experienced symptoms related to this for quite some time, they were not unusual for a middle-aged woman who did not always get to the gym regularly, and both my doctor and I had discounted them. In retrospect, he should have known better and ordered routine chest x-rays which would have picked this up earlier. It was now clear that the battle had resumed in a big way.

The nature of the struggle changed from dealing with an acute and potentially curable problem to one which would be ongoing or chronic. This was a big emotional change for me and a new level of challenge. It was compounded by the fact that my symptoms were rapidly intensifying and I needed to make another series of quick decisions.

Since planning for the future had always been a big part of my career in finance (I often developed business models that looked far out into the future), I had adopted the strategy of always having something in my "back pocket." For several years, I had followed the controversy over stem cell transplants (a form of bone marrow transplantation) and had figured that, if necessary, this would be my next move. Stem cell transplant is a term that actually describes only half of a complex treatment in which the patient is given a massive dose of chemotherapy, so powerful that it kills the rapidly growing cells of the body's immune system as well as (hopefully) the cancer cells. The stem cells have to be removed first and preserved by freezing. Miraculously, once the chemo agent washes through the body, the cells can be re-introduced into the patient's blood system. They find their way back into the bone marrow where, in almost all cases, they multiply and restore the body's ability to fight infection. Transplants had been hot news items for years due to the insurance industry's reluctance to pay for their high cost: the controversy ended when Blue Cross lost a major lawsuit over its failure to authorize one for a California woman. Sadly, she lost her life due to the delay, but her legacy paved the way for others who would follow.

My experiences in being evaluated for stem cell transplants at two local hospitals are chronicled in detail in chapter 6. I was initially rejected by the first and then accepted by the second. The fact that any facility could reject a patient was news to me and even more of a shock that two facilities within only fifty miles of each other would have such widely divergent opinions. Fortunately, Dave and I had the persistence to solicit a second opinion.

Having decided to go forward, I entered a period of waiting and preparation, which included undergoing pheresis, a procedure which involves removal and filtration of blood to extract the stem cells which are later re-infused. This is the portion of the process that is an autologous (meaning "self") donation. From conversation with the nurses and a visit to the transplant ward, I knew the procedure would be rough and was determined to do something to take my mind off of it. I decided that a new hobby was in order, something I had always wanted to pursue, but had never had time for: I would take a photography course in the two weeks I had left prior to checking into the hospital. Having made this decision, I acted immediately. As soon as the pheresis was done, I walked out of the blood filtration room and down the hospital corridor to a telephone booth. I then made three phone calls: one to the photography school in Maine that I wanted to attend, a second to book a plane flight, and a third to get a hotel room. I was in luck as everything clicked and within days I was on a plane, flying across the country accompanied only by my wig, a Hickman arterial access line inserted in my chest, and my camera. The class was terrific, Maine was inspiring, and it was refreshing to be somewhere where no one knew the challenge I had to deal with. *Constantly distracting myself with new projects became a hallmark of my coping strategy.*

Upon my return, I checked into the hospital for what proved to be a very long month's stay. The nurses had warned me that the transplant, which involves receiving a near fatal dose of chemotherapy, was one of the toughest medical procedures, second only to heart surgery. This proved to be true, although it was viewed through the haze of morphine which was administered almost constantly.

Despite my somewhat tenuous interaction with the world, I was fortunate to have an almost constant stream of visitors who dutifully made the nearly fifty-mile trek several times a week to visit. My friend Anita kept me occupied with endless games of Scrabble. Amazingly, I was even able to beat her occasionally. She now jokes that I can only win under the influence of morphine. Another friend, Joyce, adorned my room with prints of digital images she had made. A former colleague of my husband's invested a lot of time making me a beautiful quilted bed jacket which she personally delivered to the hospital. My husband, Dave, and my mother took turns sleeping on a cot in my room, so I was hardly ever alone.

In addition, I was constantly surprised by the generosity of both current and old friends. Many people came in to the hospital to donate blood and platelets, and my mother took over as the chief coordinator for these donations, telling people when and where they needed to show up. While blood donation is relatively simple, giving platelets is more involved, taking two to three hours. An old family friend I had not seen much since childhood actually drove several hours to come in for a visit as well as a donation. Another wrote almost weekly letters describing how my situation had inspired her to deal with a painful marital problem. Such support, much of it unexpected, was enormously helpful.

The majority of the time, I was not in any particular pain because of the morphine, administered by a bedside machine over which I had complete control. Despite the unpleasantness of the procedure, which wreaks havoc with your immune system, digestive tract, and blood chemistry, the pain can easily be controlled by the systemic use of morphine. Although many people (and not a few of their doctors) fear that they might become addicted to morphine or other pain killers, this rarely occurs. When the pain stops, so does the desire for morphine. Enduring pain is hardly ever a good idea and many enlightened physicians consider effective pain control a given. Although I frequently ran high fevers, I was only vaguely aware of them. I slowly realized that the ordeal was at least as difficult for my friends and family to watch as it was for me to endure and, perhaps, even more so. They often looked worried and frightened by what was going on. The ward was a difficult place to visit, since all the patients there were in the same situation. Besides the obvious illness, the intensive chemotherapy caused everyone to loose all of their hair, including eyebrows and eyelashes. I joked that we all looked like Martians. In fact, my friend Anita said she accidentally walked into the wrong room and didn't know it, since we all looked so much alike!

Some of the most difficult moments were in the middle of the night. Unable to sleep and intensely uncomfortable, I went in search of popsicles—kept in constant supply at the nurses' station to soothe the chronic mouth sores resulting from the temporary immune system suppression.

Although calm most of the time, I did have some emotional lows. One afternoon, Dave showed up in my room and I let loose with a rare outburst, shouting that this was a terrible procedure, most likely would do no good, and I should have just let the disease run its course. He began to rub my feet (a habit he had adopted to comfort me when I seemed to be inconsolable), continued to listen quietly and then asked if I had heard the news that day. It turned out that Lady Diana Spencer had been killed in an auto accident. A vibrant, healthy life was now gone, and I was still here. It made a huge impression and, ironically, helped me vow to return to life again.

Thirty days later, I left the hospital and moved in with my parents for the remaining recovery. Dave's job required much travel and I was too weak to be alone for any significant period of time. Despite my fierce independence, I was grateful I could rely on them. This period was probably more difficult than the hospital stay since I was off the drugs and more aware of all the aftereffects of the treatment. I was routinely awake in the middle of the night suffering from nausea, with my mother almost always up and standing nearby. But I had daily visits from a local nurse and gradually returned to normal. My friends continued to visit almost as much as I could allow. Nearly four months after I entered the hospital and about nine months after I stopped working, I was able to resume a consulting practice helping young companies develop their business models. Returning to work and some semblance of a normal life has always been a coping strategy for me. I had a clean set of scans and the hope that the grueling therapy might actually have cured me.

Since the stem cell had been my "back pocket" strategy, I also began looking for the next thing in case it failed. I had long been interested in clinical trials and began to review what was available in earnest. The common belief at that time was that once you had gone through a stem cell transplant, you had received a lifetime dose of toxins and your chemotherapy career was over, so I focused on looking at non-toxic therapies.

I found an interesting vaccine study being conducted at the University of Washington in Seattle for patients who over-expressed a protein called HER-2. This protein is encoded by a special type of gene called an oncogene (oncogenes are involved in controlling cell growth), called her-2[1]. It had been found that in about 30 percent of breast cancer patients, a condition arises causing this gene to be amplified (resulting in excessive activity) and/or over-expressed (resulting in too many copies of the gene). In both cases, the result is a high number of copies of the protein, which in turn drives the cell to divide abnormally. This results in cancer. The vaccine study was designed to expose patients to fragments of the protein in an attempt to get the body to develop its own immune response.

Having known about her-2, I had long ago insisted on having my original biopsy slide tested and knew that I was among the 30 percent subset. I contacted the study site and spoke with the recruitment nurse. She acknowledged that I was a candidate for the study, but also indicated that the recruitment was closed. Although initially disappointed, I vowed not to give up easily and began a campaign to call her every few weeks to check on the status. After a number of calls, an opening arose when another candidate dropped out. My persistence had again paid off and I immediately enrolled in the trial.

I began a series of trips from the Bay Area to Seattle for the injections. The nursing staff there was terrific and I had a chance to discuss the science behind the study as well as what was going on with clinical trials in general. I made a point of combining each visit, which took about two to three hours, with lunch at an

---

[1]    This nomenclature represents standard practice in medical genetics where the gene is described in lower case letters and the protein it is responsible for coding in upper case letters.

interesting restaurant or a visit to a museum or other place of interest before I returned home on a late afternoon flight.

During the fourth vaccination visit, I mentioned to the study nurse that I was experiencing a bit of tingling and numbness in my left leg. She looked concerned, and suggested that I report it to my doctor as soon as possible. When I got home, I made an appointment to see the UCSF physician I have continued to consult whenever something new pops up.

He was initially unconcerned; he thought it probably was a minor neuropathy. (Neuropathy is a general term that applies to a wide range of medical issues associated with nerve irritation.) When the symptoms persisted, I suggested that I have an MRI. He agreed to set this up, although at the time he wasn't convinced it was necessary. The day prior to the scan, I called him to suggest that we cancel it, but he urged me not to.

The technician running the MRI seemed nervous after I was finished. That evening, I received an urgent call from my doctor. The scan had showed that there was a tumor growing in my spinal cord that had the ability to cause paralysis if it was not treated immediately. He prescribed medication to reduce the swelling, scheduled additional MRIs, and set me up for a radiation consultation the next day. In just a short period of time, I was back in the middle of treatment, and it was more serious than it had ever been.

I met with a radiologist the very next morning.

"I'm amazed that you caught this so quickly," she said. "We usually don't see people until they are almost completely paralyzed on one side. At that point, it's unusual for us to be able to see much of a recovery."

Unfortunately, another set of MRIs showed that I also had a small lesion in the back of my brain. It was only a minor comfort that our friend Brian, a professor at Stanford University who does research on brain function, noted that it's an area that "doesn't do very much. In fact, we're not sure it does anything."

The double whammy meant that I was in for a dual course of radiation, one set to my spine and another to my brain. Due to a concern that there might be microscopic brain lesions, whole brain radiation was recommended.

The treatments were daily and although radiation is painless, it does generate a variety of side effects. Having your entire brain radiated is a strange experience. In addition to the customary hair loss, which I was well acquainted with from traditional chemotherapy, I experienced lightening-like flashes of light in my visual system which came and went during the radiation. Significant fatigue began almost immediately and lasted for several months. It was debilitating.

In addition to the radiation, I also contacted my physician to discuss starting a course of Herceptin®, a newly approved drug that had just been released to treat women who over-expressed the her-2 gene. While he agreed to this treatment, he advised me against having high expectations, indicating that only about 30 percent of patients responded to the drug at all, and of this subset, only 10 percent had truly dramatic results. This meant that my chances for a remission were somewhere in the 3 percent range overall. Having tracked the development of this drug, I was a firm believer in the therapy. To his surprise, I experienced dramatic improvement after just two doses of Herceptin®.

About halfway through the radiation, I began having blood chemistry problems, in particular with my platelet counts. Platelets are responsible for causing blood clotting when you have a wound, and the low platelet count put me at serious risk not only because of the possibility of uncontrolled bleeding from an external cut but to increased risk of internal bleeding and stroke. Things were looking bleak.

In an attempt to stabilize the blood chemistry, I had several platelet transfusions, but my body either rejected the platelets outright or chewed them up in a matter of days, so I was left with the same low counts. To my amazement, the doctors scratched their heads and said there was "nothing they could do for me." I was already experiencing light bleeding from my gums, nose and even eyes. Despite the bleeding risk, they suggested I go home and try to recover.

I was aghast and asked to be hospitalized. They refused, again saying that nothing could be done. Feeling as if I had just been thrown overboard and then had my life preserver snatched away, I went home to ponder what I would do next.

By the time I got there, I had worked myself into quite a state. As I was lying on the sofa, the room began to spin. I felt as if I was going to pass out. Somehow I had the presence of mind to unlock the front door, grab the phone, and call 911. The fire department with a paramedic team was there within minutes. They took my blood pressure, refused to tell me the result (it was over 200), then rushed me to the nearest emergency room.

My visit to the ER was a fiasco. I ended up with several incorrect diagnoses, including one suggesting that I had experienced a heart attack (I had not). At the hospital's insistence, I went to consult a cardiologist, who confirmed my own conclusion. In the end, it appeared I had suffered a panic attack, which I eventually self-diagnosed when all else proved negative. At that point, my radiologist agreed to admit me to the hospital, where I remained for the next four days.

I slowly recovered from the low platelets as well as a reduced white count, but was subjected to additional tests and misdiagnoses. The hospital assigned a physician who had a well-known and somewhat mixed reputation. When he entered my room, his first words to me were, "Didn't you participate in the television documentary on breast cancer?" I had totally forgotten that he had also been a part of the program.

The half hour show had featured three patients' stories with only about five minutes for each of us. I had decided to illustrate my point about "taking charge" by telling how I was rejected for the stem cell transplant *at the very hospital where I was now again a patient.*

Apparently, my attending physician was annoyed that I had spoken out on the show, even though I was careful not to name the institution publicly. Saying he was "sure that everyone knew who it was," he obviously viewed this as a public criticism of his hospital. He seemed to have no concern whatsoever for my perspective or for the possibility that my treatment rejection had been made in error, thus forcing me to look for an alternative. This was a particularly discouraging way to start a new relationship, even more so given the shape I was in. I must say, it was one of the low points of all my interaction with physicians and the medical establishment. Many of the former (and certainly the latter) do not respond well to criticism of any kind. Although this episode felt extreme, since I was hardly in any condition to defend myself—having a fever of 102° at the time—I encountered defensiveness and closed mindedness at odd times throughout my odyssey.

Moreover, this newest member of my team was convinced that my stem cell transplant had either failed or that I had leukemia. I believed neither and that I was merely reacting to having had too much radiation, an assessment based on all of the prior problems I had experienced recovering from other therapies which often turned out to have an excessive effect on me. I believed that my own physiology was unusually reactive to many medications and to procedures such as radiation. Despite my protests, he insisted that I undergo both a bone marrow aspiration as well as a spinal tap. Both were negative and proved that my initial instincts were correct.

Slowly, I recovered and returned for a consultation with this same oncologist. That's when we had the infamous conversation (which I cover in detail in Chapter 3: Choosing a Physician) in which he told me that there was "no benefit in treating a woman with metastatic breast cancer," and that he would not offer me any treatment with Herceptin®, due to his belief that it was the culprit in my blood chemistry problems. This was one of the most negative meetings I have ever experienced. I walked out of his office, never to return.

In desperation, I contacted my physician at UCSF and asked for a referral to someone more compatible. He immediately set me up with a doctor who was part of a private practice in Campbell, only a few miles from my home. The first visit confirmed that this was the right place for me: a small group of physicians who ran their own show; a cracker-jack nursing team; receptionists who actually smiled and seemed to know everyone's name; and even an in-house lab that could crank out blood chemistry results in five minutes.

We resumed treatment with Herceptin® on an every-other-week basis. About two months into this, I asked to be re-scanned utilizing both MRI and CT. Anyone who has undergone scanning knows that although the procedure itself is painless, there is much anxiety associated with waiting for the results. I had gotten into the habit of pestering the technicians to show me the scans while they were still up on the screen. This was clearly against hospital policy—probably for good reasons, since most patients will panic if given bad news with no one to talk to immediately, as well as the fact that proper interpretation of these kinds of scans is not particularly intuitive.

My strategy this time was to befriend the technician (luckily, I was assigned a woman) who was conducting the MRI. This scan would reveal whether the most serious of the tumors, those in the brain and spinal cord, had changed. When I got up from the table, I casually walked over to her, let her know my history, and asked if she could tell me whether the tumors were smaller or larger. She frowned, puzzled, and then, noting that she was not a radiologist, asked where they were.

"I really don't see anything that looks like a tumor," she said.

Amazed, we quickly looked at all of the scans and failed to find even the smallest remnant of tumor. I went home elated! A subsequent CT scan showed that I was clean in other less critical areas as well.

I had made nothing less than a miraculous recovery, all based on the therapy with Herceptin®. I soon found out that although up to 30 percent of breast cancer patients respond somewhat to Herceptin®, the remission I had achieved was shared by only about 3 percent of patients. I felt like the new poster girl for the drug.

I continued treatment on a bi-monthly basis and resumed my consulting practice. As I grew confident that my illness was under control (perhaps even cured?) I accepted a full-time senior management position with a newly formed company, Shutterfly.com, in the emerging market of digital photography. Life seemed to once again resume a semblance of normalcy.

My health continued to be happily uneventful for almost two years. Then a routine chest x-ray revealed a small shadow in my lung. CT and MRI scans confirmed that the tumors had re-grown in all of the previously affected areas. When and how quickly this had happened was a mystery, since we had not been doing routine scans.

This third and latest recurrence has proven to be the most difficult emotionally. Clearly, the cure I had hoped for had not materialized and I was forced to come to terms with the fact that I would be living with this disease on an on-going basis. I needed to get used to this and decided to step out of the workforce unless I could achieve another remission, which seemed unlikely.

Once again, the immediate focus was on the brain and spinal cord, where the lesions had the most potential for disastrous impact. The MRI had revealed that there were two brain lesions now, the original tumor which had re-grown and a tiny new one. I started to look into novel therapies.

Through my network of cancer friends as well as the advice of my radiation oncologist, I was steered towards a treatment at Stanford Medical Center which was still experimental and had been used on only a few hundred patients. Known as the CyberKnife®, it was a non-invasive form of radiosurgery which has the ability to target tumors with extreme accuracy to within a 1mm error. An advance over conventional radiotherapy, which involves radiating an entire field, the CyberKnife® can deliver a therapeutic dose directly to the tumor site, leaving adjacent tissue unaffected.

The CyberKnife® was a clear advance over an older technology, known as the Gamma Knife, which can also target a small area. Unlike the CyberKnife®, however, it had no automatic feedback loop to correct for head movement during radiation delivery. Without this corrective ability, patients are forced to wear an uncomfortable head-mounted stabilization device which literally has to be bolted to their skulls to inhibit head movement. A quick peek at the head frame convinced me that the CyberKnife® therapy would be the better choice.

However, I was disturbed to discover that the CyberKnife® was about to be dismantled for a software upgrade and would be out-of-order for almost six months. I had to use every tactic at my disposal to convince the hospital to squeeze me into the schedule before the equipment went down. This included daily phone calls and reaching out to other contacts I had made both in the hospital as well as the associated teaching facility.

I underwent the CyberKnife® during the summer of 2001 and was amazed by how easy and painless it was. Fascinated by the technology, I actually went back and interviewed the radiology team as well a representative of the company that had developed the equipment. The article I wrote was published in a local breast cancer newsletter and is included in Chapter 7: Emerging Therapies.

In addition to the CyberKnife®, I underwent additional radiation to my spine. Unfortunately, the spinal cord is limited in terms of the maximum radiation that can be tolerated, so I was only able to undergo a few treatments. Nevertheless, subsequent scans have shown that the tumor had either shrunk or shown no new activity.

Following the radiation, I resumed chemotherapy with an initial regimen that combined Herceptin® and Taxol®. I lost my hair for the fifth time—an event I was well acquainted with, but never had quite gotten used to. I also suffered from fatigue, a common complaint of chemo patients.

Things were stable for about seven months when new scans reflected growth in a few areas. At that point, we switched to a combination of Navelbine® and Herceptin® which kept the cancer dormant for another six months. Finally, after about a year, a new CT scan reflected some alarming growth in a liver lesion, which required us to leap back into action.

Fortunately, I had briefly looked into another "back pocket" strategy. Radio Frequency (RF) ablation had shown good success in treating liver problems. In fact, I had already suggested this to both of my medical advisors who believed that we should wait for further change before proceeding. With the remaining areas still dormant, the time was now.

A relatively new technique, RF ablation is a laparoscopic procedure which treats the lesion directly with heat to kill a selected area of tissue (known as "ablation"). Laparoscopic means that the entire surgery is done without a traditional incision, guided by a miniature TV camera. Both the camera and the other instruments are inserted through mini-incisions. One of the wonders of modern surgical technique, laparoscopy results in much less trauma, much faster healing and quicker recovery for the patient. I jokingly referred to this as my "foie gras" treatment since it essentially involved cooking a small piece of the liver with a probe. Only a few physicians in the Bay Area perform this procedure; I was fortunate enough to be steered towards a very experienced young doctor at UCSF. My first call to his office got me booked three weeks later for an evaluation. However, since my tumor was on the threshold of what they considered treatable (less than 5 cm), I thought it was imperative that the surgery happen quickly. I worked on enlisting the nurse's sympathy in order to accelerate this appointment. Dave and I ended up in his office a week later.

As we waited for the surgeon, the nurse greeted us with a warning that we not be alarmed by the surgeon's youthful appearance (medicine seems to be the one area where age discrimination works in reverse), and assured us that the "older doctors really can't learn to do this procedure. You have to be good at video games to do complicated laparoscopic surgery."

With that prelude, the surgeon arrived and put up the CT scans. Dave and I were shocked by both the increase and overall size of the lesion. It's an odd experience, but the ability to visually see the enemy is both frightening and empowering.

"I had wanted to come and see you earlier," I said, "when the tumor was a bit smaller. But both of my doctors said we should wait and that this procedure could be done in the future."

He confirmed that it would have been preferable for me to have come in earlier and acted surprised that my team hadn't acted more aggressively. Fortunately, he concluded that the lesion could still be treated using laparoscopy, which meant I would be spared from a much larger and more complicated surgery.

With some additional negotiation, the surgery was scheduled for the following week and I was able to breathe a big sigh of relief. The operation went as planned and required only an overnight stay at the hospital. The recovery, however, was much tougher than expected. I spent the first week almost entirely in bed; the second, moving from the bed to the sofa and back, and the third and fourth weeks making short forays out into the world. It turned out to be a particularly painful time, eased primarily by the fact that the surgery was believed to have been successful. I had bought another chunk of time.

Everything went well until a new scan four months later indicated that we had not gotten everything and that there was still residual tumor. Much to my dismay, I had to undergo a second procedure in November of that year, which necessitated the same difficult recovery all over again.

After breathing another sigh of relief that this was over, I was faced with yet another challenge in early December. A follow-up MRI scan showed that the brain lesion that had been treated with the CyberKnife appeared to be enlarging and was also surrounded by edema (excessive fluid retention), which was causing some swelling. Surprisingly, despite all of this change in my brain tissue, I was asymptomatic. We ran a second (spectroscopic) MRI to measure the metabolic activity of that area of the brain to discern whether this was an active tumor or just an artifact of the radiation treatment. Unfortunately, the test was inconclusive, leaving me with the decision of whether or not to operate. It was only two weeks before Christmas.

The notion of brain surgery was a bit daunting—even after all of the other therapy I had been through. I remember asking the surgeon to rate the difficulty and risks associated with this operation on a scale of one to ten (with ten being the most serious). He said it was a "two" and that I could either wait and see what else developed, or go in now with the least risk of complications.

I was fortunate that my friend Joyce had accompanied me to the meeting with my neurosurgeon. She listened carefully, asked a lot of good questions, and when it was over, helped me arrive at my final decision. I have often found it useful to have a second pair of ears along when consulting with physicians or other diagnosticians. These discussions can be stress producing, if not frightening. It helps to have someone listen who is at least slightly less involved. Obviously, one should choose a friend or companion who is a good and constructive listener. It didn't take me long to decide to go ahead. The lesion was just under the surface of my skull and, even though this involved cutting out a piece of the bone (which was later put back in place with small titanium screws), it was easily accessible. The risk of permanent damage was almost nil.

The surgery was scheduled for just over a week later and, in fact, I had it the day after my husband and I hosted a Christmas party at our home for forty people. Although not everyone knew what I would be facing the next morning, those who did were amazed that I would go ahead with the party. It turned out to be a great distraction and I could think of no better thing to do the day before a major operation. The room was filled with love and support.

The surgery ended up being much more difficult from a psychological point of view than a physical one. The preparation involved shaving several small areas on my head and attaching electrodes which would be used to monitor brain function during the surgery and provide "calibration points" on the skull so that the neurosurgeon could keep track of the exact location of the lesions. I also had to undergo another CT scan just prior to the operation so that the exact location could be marked and sent to the operating room, where it was used to actually guide the surgery through an imaging technology. Insisting on being conscious for the ride to the OR—I felt like I probably looked like the bride of Frankenstein when they wheeled me in—I asked a few questions about the equipment and then decided I didn't need to know too much more. They put me out with a few long breaths of gas.

I awoke in the intensive care unit suffering from only a mild headache and a bit less hair. In general, so little hair had to be sacrificed (due to the "vanity cuts" that are now routinely performed) that for many patients, it is not even visible. Several friends soon came by to visit, including my friend Lucy. She later told me that she approached my room with some trepidation, not knowing what shape I would be in. She was surprised to find me sitting up in bed, talking and making jokes. Even the OR nurse said she "wasn't used to patients being so mobile in the ICU."

With no apparent problems, I transferred to a regular room for an additional night and went home the next morning. As I now tell everyone, the "brain surgery was the easy part."

I did suffer one rather disturbing side effect that the neurosurgeon now believes was due to post-surgical swelling. The lesion and associated swelling had been near one of the brain's visual centers and I had great difficulty with reading for about two months afterwards. Everything slowed down to the point that I could only process about four letters at a time, making even simple reading a major chore. Interestingly, my brain researcher friend Brian was able to explain to me what was going on. Apparently, the area of the brain that was affected is responsible for learned language and I was suffering from "alexia without agraphia." Translated into terms I could understand, this meant that I was able to process only a small reading window at a time. Apparently when we read, we normally only see about four letters concurrently, but are able to scan quickly and also make educated guesses about what will come next to speed the brain's processing of information. In my brain, this whole complex process had slowed down. Interestingly, however, I did not have this problem with writing and reading my own words (known as agraphia). I must admit that although the scientific explanation was fascinating, it was very disturbing to wake up one morning and be so acutely aware that something in my brain was not functioning quite the way it had just the previous day. Fortunately, I recovered slowly over the next several months with no residual effects.

The really good news is that the follow-up brain biopsy indicated no active tumor and only a residual necrosis (i.e., dying tissue) which had resulted from the CyberKnife treatment. The therapy had obviously worked, and although the surgery had not in hindsight been absolutely necessary, it was a relief to have gotten it over with and have a clear answer.

Just a month later, there was equally good news from a follow-up CT scan which showed that the liver lesion was now completely gone. I was down to only one site (lungs) which contained lesions, and these were relatively stable.

Although I'm not cured, I clearly have the upper hand at the moment. The goal now is managing and living with this as long as possible. At my chemotherapy visit this past week, I announced to my doctor that I was celebrating my ten-year anniversary as a survivor. I said to him, "Let's go for another ten years."

His response: "Why not twenty?"

# Chapter 2

## Getting the Correct Diagnosis

Nearly everyone can understand the trauma associated with receiving a diagnosis of a serious illness. Like many of life's dramatic moments, the time, the place, the words are instantly fixed in memory. Less obvious, however, is the fact that getting a *correct* diagnosis can often be the patients' first challenge.

Many serious illnesses start with relatively benign symptoms and vague complaints which are often associated with minor ailments. A patient who presents to a doctor and fits a profile for a specific illness will often be given a screening test for the ailment, but such tests are not always 100 percent effective at detecting underlying conditions. More sophisticated tests are often deemed unwarranted due to cost (such as CT scans and MRIs) and/or the patients' age.

I was initially misdiagnosed. I went to see my primary care practitioner after noticing pain during my regular weight-lifting workouts. It felt as if a small, pea-sized pebble was pressing against my chest directly beneath my left breast. The pain was apparent in certain positions and was consistent over time. My first meeting with the doctor resulted in a mammogram and an exam, both negative. I went away with a sense of relief, only to continue experiencing the same symptoms. At the urging of my husband, Dave, I returned to my doctor a month later with the same complaint. She did a repeat of the physical exam, but said she saw "no reason" for another mammogram. I was uneasy with her conclusion and told her so. Reluctantly, she said I "could get another opinion" if I really wanted to.

I have a very clear memory of this moment, as I looked her in the eye and asked, "Do I need one?" Some part of me realized that I was putting an awful lot of faith in her response, faith that I might regret in the future. She seemed young and somewhat inexperienced. My intuition was telling me that there was something wrong and, in fact, this was the first time I had ever directly challenged a physicians' judgment. I had also always been the kind of person who plans for the "downside" in life, and was used to thinking through all of the possible outcomes related to every situation. All of this was directly at odds with my desire to hear good news. So, when my doctor replied, "No, you don't need a second opinion," I accepted this answer against my better judgment. After all, this was the answer I had wanted to hear, reinforced by the fact that I had no family history of breast cancer, no known risk factors, and was still quite young, only 38. All of this was noted by the doctor and recorded with her comments in my medical record.

Five months later, I awoke one morning to find a lump protruding from the side of my left breast. It had not been visible or even palpable before. Realizing that my discomfort with my family practitioner had been well-founded and concerned about the delay, I immediately scheduled a consultation with a surgeon. To my surprise, he was very blasé, indicating that the lump was probably benign; I should schedule a biopsy, to be sure, but there was no urgency. My response was immediate and firm, "How about tomorrow?" This was the first of many steps towards taking control of my medical destiny. He was taken aback, but acquiesced when I insisted. I was not interested in wasting any more time dealing with what I was now convinced was a serious problem. I had the biopsy the next day.

It's not clear why, but it can take up to a week to receive the results of a biopsy. During this time, most people are on pins and needles and I certainly was nervous and on edge. Several days passed before the phone rang in my office at work. The surgeon was abrupt and to the point. "It's cancer," he said. "You need to have immediate surgery." I think I mumbled something about "talking about this," made a quick appointment and hung up the phone. In the midst of this, someone had walked into my office and was horrified by the expression on my face. I was speechless for several minutes and then made a mad dash for the ladies room. A nearby colleague, sensing something was quite amiss, followed me to offer support.

After calming down, I made my way downtown to the appointment I had just insisted on with the surgeon. He gave me a lot of information, much of which went in one ear and out the other: I was still in shock. The difficulty of processing information while you are upset is compounded by the fact that many illnesses force you to make decisions—which may or may not be essential—in a fairly short timeframe. With cancer, the convention within the medical profession is to remove the offending lesion with the utmost haste, lest it spread to other parts of the body. The truth is, many cancers have been resident for several years (some experts claim up to eight years) prior to being detected. A delay of several weeks is unlikely to change the ultimate outcome and will enable the patient to become sufficiently informed so he or she can play an active part in the process. The belief that treatment must always begin immediately is just one of many myths in medicine which are surprisingly slow to change.

With breast cancer, I soon learned that mammograms have about a 30 percent false negative in young women (i.e., about 30 percent of the time, a young woman who actually has breast cancer will have a negative mammogram). This is because breast tissue in young women can be quite dense and mask the appearance of a tumor. At 38, I unfortunately fell into this category. Physical exams for cancer can detect a lesion only when it gets to about 2.5cm (one inch) in size, at which point it is beyond the initial stage (cancers are typically staged from I to IV according to size and spread to other parts of the body). A doctor relying on a negative mammogram and a negative physical exam, despite protestations from the patient, can still come up with a misdiagnosis. Patients need to rely on their own intuition when things don't seem right—

if something feels wrong, insist on additional testing and don't take no for an answer.

Another even more alarming situation involved my mother. Unbelievably, she also began battling breast cancer just a short time after my own diagnosis. Luckily, hers was detected early and she has avoided any recurrence problems thus far. This was far from a simple process.

We were now both patients of the same clinic. My mother went to visit her physician for a routine mammogram about a year after my own problem surfaced. Unfortunately, the mammogram showed a suspicious area in one breast, subsequently confirmed as cancer by a biopsy.

After much angst and debate, she checked into the hospital for surgery which was uneventful and spent a painful several weeks recovering at home. However, given my misdiagnosis at this same clinic, I was uncomfortable. I insisted that she visit my new radiologist/mammographer, who I believed to be the top person in the Bay Area, so she could review the treatment my mom had received.

My mother's initial reaction was to resist, insisting that everything was OK, and that the rest of the family was comfortable with the results. Her reluctance caused me to take an unusually strong position.

"Your life is on the line here," I said simply and forcefully. "I insist that you to see this physician immediately!"

Surprised by my outburst, my mother made an appointment and brought along the mammography films from the other clinic. The radiologist reviewed them and immediately asked, "Didn't they say anything about the other breast?" My mother had been told there were no other problems and to come back in a year for a routine check. The new physician insisted on an immediate biopsy and found a second cancer on the other side, which was much more aggressive than the first and would have become invasive if left untreated for another year. Mom was back in the hospital for surgery within weeks of the initial procedure. I was relieved that she left our old clinic for good, especially when I later found out that another good friend's mother had been misdiagnosed by the same clinic and died as a result of delayed treatment.

Several years later, I invited this radiologist to participate as a speaker at a seminar I had organized on breast cancer. I had the emotional and extraordinary pleasure of introducing her as the woman who saved my mother's life.

I cannot stress enough the importance of pushing for an accurate and rapid diagnosis. Patients should be aware of the full range of diagnostic tests available when basic screening tests do not adequately answer important questions. With breast cancer, traditional mammography leaves a lot to be desired. In fact, the routine screening of women beginning at age forty has been quite a controversial topic over the past several years due to both the cost as well as the unknown benefits to younger women. I was unaware at the time that ultrasound, a much more sensitive test, could possibly have detected my problem earlier, as could CT and MRI scans. Unfortunately they are all much more expensive than a mammogram.

Anyone suspicious that she has not had an adequate diagnostic workup should be careful to quiz the doctor about other tests that may exist, and then insist on them if she is not satisfied. Since physicians are sometimes reluctant to order expensive tests when they are not convinced they are truly warranted, this may require some patient assertiveness. A friend/advocate can help take some of the emotion out of the interaction. Failing this, you can always get another doctor.

We all want a physician to reassure us that there is nothing wrong and nothing to worry about. But there may be a high price to pay for hearing only what you want. It is always a good idea to find a doctor who is cautious, performs comprehensive tests and wants to be sure.

I will never know if the initial six-month delay in my diagnosis was responsible for my ongoing fight with cancer, but the realization that it *could be* certainly created my resolve to take charge of and manage the process right from the beginning.

# Processing Initial Information

Once I had a diagnosis in hand, there was a deluge of information to sort through in a very short time. The medical profession has clearly made attempts to provide literature and some minimal patient education. However, much of this is just the bare basics and does not provide adequate tools for evaluating complex treatment options.

There is a method for absorbing information and it's best to begin at a general level. I made the mistake of showing up at the Stanford University Medical School Library on Day Two to search the medical archives for technical articles. I was overwhelmed by detailed scientific research into obscure topics and sidelines. And I was equally horrified by decades-old photos of women with total mastectomies which in the earlier days were much more disfiguring due to the removal of the underlying muscle (a procedure which is rarely done today). A better start would have been to read a good overview of breast cancer, like *Dr. Susan Love's Breast Book*[2].

For patients who have an interest in basic medical research, it is possible to find someone who is well-versed in the literature and will offer to meet on a consulting basis to explain the history of various treatments and likely outcomes. They can most often be found in university settings, where they combine both research and clinical careers. Through a local breast cancer support group, Dave and I were able to find Dr. Craig Henderson at a local university, a well-regarded and widely known breast cancer researcher. He spent almost two hours with us going over all of the research on chemotherapy and survival rates. When we left his office, we both felt we had a good foundation in the basic research and enough information to make treatment decisions. Although what we learned about treatment options was no different from what my oncologist had told us, the additional research information

---

[2]    Love, Dr. Susan and Lindsey, Karen, *Dr. Susan Love's Breast Book*, Addison Wesley Publishers, 1995

gave us a heightened degree of confidence and understanding of the disease.

Talking to fellow patients can also be helpful, although the experience and background of others may be significantly different. Nevertheless, it is always comforting to speak to someone who has not only survived, but even thrived following a breast cancer diagnosis (see more on this in Chapter 4). When I announced my condition to a women's group I was part of, I was almost immediately inundated with referrals to fellow breast cancer survivors. They proved to be an enormous source of support, encouragement and hope. I'll never forget one early conversation I had with a woman in her sixties who described her experience with breast reconstruction.

"Well," she said, "when I had my reconstructive surgery I made a decision to augment the remaining breast. I decided that if I had to go through all of this, I wanted to get something out of it. Now I look better in a bathing suit than I ever did!" The fact that she had survived and could look on the bright side made me feel infinitely better.

I found several things about the early learning process to be quite stressful. First and foremost, you are faced with the task of processing an enormous amount of information in a short period of time, during which you are still adjusting to the initial shock of being told you have a life-threatening disease. In addition, you are not the only one processing information: you must deal with the reactions of your friends and family, and their struggle in coming to terms not only with your challenge but with their own mortality. This feels a bit like being dropped in the middle of a battle-zone with no weapons and no training.

When dealing with an illness like cancer, for which there is no sure cure, there are a multitude of options and approaches, ranging from surgery only to highly toxic forms of chemotherapy to radiotherapy and to multiple clinical trials. As an initial treatment, physicians tend to recommend what they are familiar with and what has a history of practice. I think of this as "cookbook" medicine, where a specific set of parameters dictates a specific therapy.

Although we would all like to think of ourselves as individuals, and our therapy as specific to our individual bodies, most medicine is based on mathematical population "averages," which do not take into account individual differences. Chemotherapy, for example, is a given drug administered according to a treatment protocol which has been shown to be effective for the average patient. Drug dosage is based on body weight and volume and the duration of treatment is based on results from clinical trials. Rudimentary statistics imply that while this dose may be fine for the average person, it will be too much for some and perhaps too little for others. Moreover, there has been no systematic attempt to test tumor samples for susceptibility to specific drugs. Recent developments, however, in the biotech field have pointed to a future which might include genetic testing of biopsy samples to determine which drugs might be most effective for a given patient's tumor. Genomic Health, a company located in Redwood City, California, is currently leading the way in this new field.

Only now, with the sequencing of the human genome, the code of life, is the medical profession beginning to talk about therapies that in the future can be specifically tailored to the genetic profile of a unique individual.

I quickly learned that there will be a multitude of opinions, and getting a second opinion will not always make the decision process easier. Since physicians are trained to take control, they tend to convey decisiveness and confidence that is not always warranted. During the course of my treatment, I challenged several physicians on this point. One of them, in an unusually candid moment, asked me if he should "be honest with patients about how much the medical profession really doesn't know." The fact is that many patients don't really *want* to know and prefer to put their trust and lives in the hands of a doctor who will simply tell them what to do. The medical system in this country encourages this transfer of control from the patient to the physician. For some, this may be the only choice, but I believe it increases the risk of a negative outcome.

Information overload coupled with the emotion inherent in dealing with the crisis at hand means that all but the sturdiest individuals will occasionally experience what can only be characterized as numbness. This can vary from inability to concentrate to outright confusion. It can be very helpful if someone close to the patient accompanies her on medical appointments and assists with research, if only to take notes so that a clear record of the meeting/information exists. Some people recommend using a tape recorder so that the focus can be on the conversation instead of note-taking. Dave accompanied me to all of my initial consultations.

In the end, every patient needs to keep in mind that she is the one who has to go through the treatment process and live with the result. While some people opt for the most aggressive therapy possible, others will want less. The key is to make an informed choice.

## Key Insights: Getting the Correct Diagnosis

- Listen to the signals your body is giving you and continue to push for a clear diagnosis.
- If you are not satisfied, seek another opinion rather than waiting for new symptoms to emerge.
- Be sure to educate yourself about the range of diagnostic tests available for your symptoms and insist on more sophisticated and expensive tests if you are not comfortable with the initial conclusion. Ask your doctor about other tests that may be available.
- If your physician resists additional tests, enlist a friend as an advocate to argue on your behalf. If this fails, seek another opinion.
- Accept support/help when confronted with the need to learn about your illness rapidly. Four ears are better than two when dealing with the early stages of information gathering. Take a spouse or good friend along to consultations.

- Realize that opinions on treatment will vary when dealing with illnesses for which there is no one cure available.
- Resist the urge to give up control. Trust your own instincts!

# Chapter 3

## Choosing a Physician

My vision of the ideal doctor is someone whom I can trust and with whom I can work and make joint decisions. Over the past ten years, I have consulted and fired more than a half dozen physicians for a variety of reasons ranging from their refusal to consider new therapies to being unnecessarily pessimistic. Although my approach may seem a bit idiosyncratic, I believe it has played a major role in my survival. Even more unorthodox, I actually had two physicians for a period of time. One I considered my strategist, someone I always consulted for a second opinion as new challenges arose. The other physician was my day-to-day doctor who administered my ongoing therapy. Both of them are true partners who do not feel threatened by each other and together we brainstorm and discuss various ideas every time we meet. They also have great senses of humor, which can sometimes be the best medicine. Finding them was more of a challenge than I had ever imagined.

## The Art of Medicine

It is often said that medicine is an art and not a science; I believe there is more truth in that than might make many people comfortable. In fact, although it is based on fundamental biological and physiological principles, the practice of modern medicine is only about one hundred years old and relies heavily on what has worked in the past, modified only by the patient's or doctor's judgment. Changes in treatment are slow to be adopted outside of major medical centers, as are the underlying philosophies of how best to approach different situations, not the least because one of the goals of medical schools is to train physicians to behave in a similar way. While this has an obvious advantage for minor ailments, it is not necessarily advantageous with more serious conditions where sensitivity to change and rapid adaptation to new approaches may be to the patient's benefit.

One of the most glaring examples of this has been the controversy over mastectomy vs. lumpectomy for breast cancer. Until the last decade, it was common practice for a woman to enter a hospital for a breast cancer biopsy and wake up from the surgery to find her breast missing without having had the opportunity for any additional consultation or decision-making. This rather brutal approach was based on the philosophy that the cancer had to be removed immediately before it could spread to other parts of the body. In fact, most discovered cancers have been growing for an extended period of time and, in all but a few cases, a delay of days or even weeks would rarely have any effect on the final outcome. It was not until women's groups became actively involved in protesting this routine that it disappeared and was replaced by a two-step process, which involved the patient in the ultimate decision of whether to remove the breast or not.

Recently, the issue of lumpectomy (removal of a small portion of the breast tissue as opposed to the entire breast) vs. mastectomy has displaced the earlier controversy, with some doctors insisting that a woman should have the entire breast removed in order to have the best possible chance at survival, while others favor the more cosmetically and emotionally acceptable approach of a limited surgery. In fact, some doctors have shown good success with chemotherapy first, followed by an even smaller surgery after the initial tumor has been reduced. Although research has demonstrated that in most cases, the medical outcomes of lumpectomy vs. mastectomy are equivalent, many doctors continue to press for mastectomy, based largely on what has worked in the past.

A recent study at one US hospital found that only 46 percent of female patients coming in for a second opinion had been given information on all of their surgical options, and that 20 percent changed their treatment decisions based on the second opinion[3]. Of a total of 231 patients surveyed, 31 patients who were eligible for breast-conserving treatment were not offered this option. According to Dr. Monica Morrow of Northwestern University in Chicago, most women with Stage I or II breast cancer are in fact eligible for breast-sparing surgery, although national data suggest that far fewer women actually receive it.

Given the recommendation for a mastectomy, a woman may find it difficult to choose a different path since she is often made to feel that she is risking her life by making the wrong decision. Even more of a concern is the recent trend towards prophylactic mastectomy, which is done prior to any diagnosis of breast cancer. While this is typically done at the patient's request, it reveals the powerful role that fear plays with respect to cancer treatment.

It is important to keep in mind the strong bias in medicine to stick with known approaches and the reluctance to accept change. In the end, *you* will have to live with the final result.

## *Finding a Doctor: Partnership vs. Paternalism*

Until relatively recently, the predominant attitude towards patients has been paternalistic, especially with respect to serious illness. I think of this as the "Marcus Welby, M.D." approach to medicine. Many patients do not really want to know all of the details of their illness and treatment and feel more comfortable shifting that responsibility to an omniscient physician who will somehow make everything right. I believe this has worked to the disadvantage of both sides; the physician has been given the responsibility for the most serious of decisions and the patient has relinquished it to someone with no direct stake in the outcome. This highly asymmetric relationship, coupled with the imperfect

---

[3]    Norton, Amy *Second Opinion Often Shifts Breast Cancer Care*, Reuters Health, Mar. 12, 2002

nature of medicine, often leads to lawsuits when the outcome is unhappy.

I believe that a more natural and more effective approach is for both sides to realize that a good doctor-patient relationship is a partnership with equal give and take. Patients must also come to realize that they bear the ultimate responsibility and consequences, good or bad. The ultimate truth is that *no one* has as much invested in the outcome as the patient.

I have struggled with this issue during my entire ten years of treatment and have only within the past several years found a team of doctors who have been willing to accept the partnership model. This approach is not for the faint of heart, as it goes against the grain of many physicians still in practice. Anecdotes about recalcitrant doctors are scattered throughout this book: their behavior ranges from simply being difficult to actively discouraging or even withholding potential treatments. The resistance stems partly from their medical school training, which encourages them to take charge, and from a reluctance to admit that many medical decisions are made with a good deal of ambiguity about the outcome. Also at issue are the many constraints within which medicine must operate (see more on this in Chapter 5).

In the end, being a true partner cedes some control to the patient which can be empowering in a situation that typically feels completely out-of-control. While the ultimate outcome cannot be guaranteed, management of the process and choices are accessible to anyone who wants them.

## Finding a Doctor: Research vs. Clinical Practice

Selecting a doctor is perhaps one of the most daunting prospects for a newly diagnosed patient. A combination of factors, including specific knowledge and experience with the illness at hand, bedside manner, access to hospital facilities and willingness to work with the patient as well as other doctors, all come into play.

I did what most of you will do—I went to see the first oncologist who was referred to me by my biopsy surgeon. Although she did an adequate job, in hindsight, I would have argued for a different course of treatment. It seems clear now that she had relatively little knowledge about newer therapies and even less inclination to use them.

New patients are usually unaware of the dividing line between research and practice, which can be critical when dealing with chronic illnesses. Clinical practice involves the application of treatments which have been developed, tested and proven over time to have specific effects on a given illness in a given stage of development. Researchers constantly strive to find new treatments that are both more effective and less toxic or otherwise harmful to the patient. The research environment is where new approaches are examined for effectiveness on small groups of patients with clinical refinement left to later stages. Many promising treatments don't pan out when subjected to rigorous human testing. Surprisingly, there is not only little crossover and communication between these two very different environments, there is a lot of rivalry.

Clinical physicians often believe that researchers are out-of-touch with the reality of daily patient care: days are filled with patient appointments, the details of running a medical office and the frustration of dealing with insurance companies. Most physicians literally do not have time to educate themselves about all of the latest drugs and therapies that are constantly undergoing evaluation. I also believe that many of them have come to resent patients' expectations that they be up to date on new therapies in addition to all of their other responsibilities. At least one of my physicians remarked that clinical trials (which can be a patient's last resort) were a "waste of time," and that "many patients spend their remaining time and money flying around the country in a futile attempt to find the elusive cure." While I liked him in many ways, he knew little about ongoing trials and he rapidly concluded after my second recurrence that there was little that medicine had to offer me. That was over five years ago. I was clearly on my own as far as trials were concerned.

Researchers, however, tend to look critically at practicing physicians as technicians who can follow a cookbook approach to treatment, but do not have the creativity and scientific training to discover new therapies or to apply old ones in creative ways. And, of course, there is always the specter of malpractice and/or litigation for the physician who strays too far from "acceptable practice." This conservatism is predictable.

In fact, there is much to be gained from encouraging these two quite different groups to come together. Professional conferences encourage dialogue and there are specific programs to facilitate a more rapid transfer of technology from research to practice. SPORE (Specialized Program of Research Excellence), for example, at UCSF, targets breast cancer. Stanford Medical Center has begun building a new state-of-the-art cancer center and a focus on what has become known as translational medicine (moving new therapies quickly from the bench to the clinic) is one of its key objectives. Overall, however, efficient communication and collaboration between the two groups remains a goal rather than a reality.

In my view, one of the most important qualifications of the ideal physician would be to have one leg in the clinic and the other in the research lab. Such practitioners do exist, although they are difficult to find: they are most often associated with large university medical centers, which foster both research and practice. Often overbooked, they struggle with the need to keep their knowledge base up to date, sponsor research of their own and deal with daily patient requirements. It is worthwhile to search for these rare individuals and to hold on tight when you find one. Through a combination of research—good sources are local breast cancer organizations and the survivor groups they sponsor—and networking, I have managed to locate one of these unusual physicians at a local research university. Although he is too far away for weekly treatments, he remains my advisor when new problems emerge.

## Finding a Doctor: Flexibility and Willingness to Work with Other Physicians

Another critical attribute is a doctor's openness to considering new approaches, both for trying new treatments as well as maintaining a collaborative attitude towards working with other physicians and specialists.

One of the most dramatic experiences I had was with a prominent physician (who was also a researcher, meeting my number one criterion) at a well-known university medical center in my area. He was assigned to me by the hospital following a second cancer recurrence just thirteen months after I had gone through a stem cell transplant. I knew his name as well as his reputation for being difficult and I was a bit concerned about working with him. I had undergone some grueling radiation to both my spine and head, which left me with a much weakened immune system (a condition known as neutropenia) and an almost complete failure to produce blood platelets, required for blood clotting, and white blood cells needed to fight infection. I had been hospitalized because of the potential for spontaneous bleeding and uncontrolled infection, so I was in no position to argue or negotiate with the hospital over their choice of doctor.

Prior to this turn of events, I had been placed on Herceptin®, a wonder drug in a new class of compounds called monoclonal antibodies. The fascinating development of this drug is detailed in a book called *Her-2*[4]. I would strongly recommend it to anyone interested in how new drugs are invented and delivered in this country. While Herceptin® is not appropriate for all types of breast cancer, for a certain class of patients it can be a miracle. The drug had been through years of clinical trials and had been FDA-approved and available openly for only about a month. I had been aware of it for several years and avidly followed its path through the FDA's clinical trials regimen. With new cancer cells popping up in various places, I had already been given a single course of treatment and had quickly demonstrated some response, but it had to be abandoned when the blood problems surfaced.

---

[4]    Bazell, Robert, *Her-2: The Making of Herceptin, a Revolutionary Treatment for Breast Cancer*, Random House, 1998

After I was released from the hospital, the doctor and I met again to discuss my ongoing treatment therapy. Due to the number of areas that were affected and my weakened health, he recommended no additional therapy. When I asked about resuming Herceptin® treatments he said he thought the drug was responsible for my reduced white cell counts and thus could not be utilized further. I argued that an equally likely culprit was all the radiation I had received, which is a known immunosuppressant, but he maintained his position and made a statement that I am sure never to forget for its arrogance, utter disregard for me and disrespect for scientific progress.

"We have data going back to 1896 that shows there is no benefit from treating a woman with metastatic breast cancer" he said. "We will just treat your symptoms as they come up."

He attempted to support this opinion by showing me a graph he had drawn to illustrate some correlation between dips in my white counts and the Herceptin® treatments.

Not quite believing what I had heard (even the intern sitting quietly in the corner looked up with surprise), I asked, "What do data going back to 1896 have to do with a drug which has been out on the market for only one month and has already shown some benefit?" I also reminded him that just because the low counts had occurred at the same time, there were other factors that could be responsible for this. It was not a foregone conclusion that Herceptin® was the problem—it could merely be a coincidence.

This only seemed to irritate him and he repeated that he would not treat me with Herceptin®. I tried another approach, which proved to be exactly the wrong one.

"Well, I have consulted another physician (someone equally well-known at a neighboring medical center who was also active in the research community), "and he believes I should give this another try."

Now he was angry. "I would bet my reputation against his any day!" he exclaimed.

I was flabbergasted by both the competitiveness that I had obviously brought out in this doctor as well as his refusal to even consider offering me any treatment option. It was, after all, *my life* we were negotiating here! So I calmly told him that I was going to pursue the option and that if he wouldn't treat me, I would find someone who would.

When he saw my resolve, he finally backed off and said he would "consider working with me on this," but demanded that I would "have to choose just one doctor." He "couldn't have me working with another physician."

Realizing that this relationship would not work, I said nothing. After several minutes, the intern became uncomfortable with the silence and suggested meekly that I go home, consider this and come back with a response the next week.

I left the clinic and never returned to see this doctor again. Since the oncologist who had suggested we resume treatment was too far away for regular visits, I asked for a referral to someone local, and that's who has been my oncologist ever since.

As I've already described, after only two months of treatment with Herceptin®, I was re-scanned in all of the affected areas and elated to discover that I had achieved a complete remission. It lasted for two years, during which I was on a maintenance regimen of Herceptin® and able to work and lead an almost completely normal life.

Although tempted, I never went back to report this happy result to the doctor who had initially refused to offer me what proved to be a life-saving treatment.

## *Finding a Doctor: Aggressiveness*

Every physician has a different idea about aggressive treatment. One of the fundamental philosophies of the Hippocratic Oath is captured in the admonition "Physicians do no harm." Most physicians take this quite seriously; however, when dealing with a life-threatening illness, there is an obvious downside to being risk-averse.

My first oncologist fell into the let's-not-make-the-patient-too-uncomfortable mindset. She prescribed a course of chemotherapy which was not the most aggressive therapy, although it was within the "standard of care" for breast cancer. I believe she did this to spare me some of the rough going associated with chemo, hoping that it would be good enough. Some of the notes she had made in my medical records (which are openly available to patients for the asking), included frequent reference to my symptoms and discomfort associated with treatment, and her hope that I would be able to complete the course. I later discovered that, given some of the characteristics of my tumor, there was a good chance that a tougher measure in the beginning would have had a much better chance for a cure and, in the final analysis, might even have spared me the recurrences. With some diseases, it's best to hit them hard before they have a chance to establish themselves. A patient's desire for aggressive therapy and the physician's willingness to provide it are definitely factors to be considered. Each patient must determine her own willingness and tolerance for aggressive rather than palliative treatment.

## Finding a Doctor: Clinical Setting

Clinical settings and patient treatment vary widely with each facility. In general, private clinics often are vastly more efficient in terms of keeping appointments, having laboratory services available on site and exhibiting heightened sensitivity to patient's time constraints. Hospitals are often at the other end of the scale, with some having developed a talent for stretching thirty-minute appointments into an entire day's affair. A lot of this has to do with the physicians' attitude, although this is influenced by infrastructure and support problems. It is fairly easy to determine how a clinic operates by observing the patients in the waiting room, as well as doing an informal survey. It's a good bet that disregard for patients' time translates into an equally casual attitude about everything else.

Attitudes towards patient care start at the top and trickle down throughout the organization: the hospital and/or clinic culture is established by values held at the highest level. In this way, medical organizations are similar to most corporations.

One of the most positive settings that I encountered was at the research hospital where I had my stem cell transplant and continue to visit for consultations. The attitude there is definitely biased towards the patient. Many of the physicians spend personal time with patient groups, and patient advocacy/feedback is encouraged. Their new cancer center maintains an educational facility with a full-time staff offering printed as well as electronic information. Educational materials are everywhere and it is easy to access information about support groups and other outside services. A friendly written policy which details the organization's dedication to patients and a "patient's bill of rights" is posted throughout, even in elevators.

I also experienced almost the opposite at a teaching hospital, where the focus seemed to be much more oriented towards the training of medical students. Waiting rooms were overcrowded, blood tests took hours to process, receptionists were unfriendly and patients were made to feel that they were lucky to be receiving any care at all. On top of this, when mistakes occurred, they seemed to be both expected and accepted. Certain departments did not appear to work well together and their competitiveness was obvious. Although I have not met the hospital administrators, I suspect that they are the source for many of these attitudinal problems.

In addition to saving time, an efficiently run clinic can be superior in terms of spotting problems which need immediate attention. For example, low white counts (neutropenia) can often result in serious, even life-threatening infections without immediate treatment. The loss of red blood cells can cause fatigue and anemia at a minimum and put serious strain on the heart if left untreated for too long. Both are relatively straightforward to treat once they are recognized. A lab which runs efficiently can spot these problems so that they can be addressed on the same day, which may prevent a small problem from becoming a more serious issue.

## Finding a Doctor: Positive Attitude

Physician attitude can have an enormous impact on the psychology of dealing with illness and the patient's own outlook towards fighting the disease. I have continued to be amazed at the amount of pessimism in medicine, particularly when dealing with the most serious of illnesses. Despite the importance of other factors, attitude has, in the end, been the primary motivator for my many decisions to change physicians.

It's not clear why, but many doctors will go out of their way to warn the patient that the prognosis is grim, the options are few and the most negative outcome is to be expected. I assume that they are doing this out of some belief that it's best to be honest up front, set realistic expectations and not give patients a false sense of hope.

This is ironic, given that there is certainly nothing to be lost and, perhaps, much to be gained by remaining optimistic about recovery.

My third oncologist seemed to have a low threshold for giving up. Following my difficult but successful recovery from a stem cell transplant (which was the treatment for my first recurrence), he informed me that we had now done "everything possible" to treat my illness, and if it arose again in the future, there would be no new options. When it did recur thirteen months later, one of the first things I did was to choose a new physician with a more optimistic attitude and more open acceptance of newly developed treatment options.

## Finding a Doctor: Firing Your Physician

I've found it necessary to fire several of my physicians. While this should not be done lightly or frequently, it is always an option.

Probably one of the more upsetting terminations was during chemotherapy following my initial diagnosis. My physician, whom I previously described as averse to aggressive treatment, suffered a personal crisis as I approached the midpoint of treatment. Overnight, she disappeared, abandoning all of her patients. The clinic, an HMO in a cost-cutting mode, assigned her full patient load to their only other oncologist, who was already running at full capacity. This was a recipe for disaster: this physician was literally running from patient to patient with appointments averaging about five minutes each.

Unfortunately for me, I developed neutropenia (low white blood counts) that resulted in a high fever. A reduction in white blood cells is a common side effect of chemotherapy, which attacks all fast growing cells in the body. Despite the fact that this was a known side effect, I had never been warned of the possibility by my physician and the initial symptoms seemed consistent with the flu. After dragging myself into the clinic, the attending doctor was so concerned that he actually drove me personally to the hospital. My cell count was so low that it was almost undetectable. The resulting hospitalization was marked by high fevers and unknown infections due to my suppressed immune system—it was touch and go for about a week. I believe that with better monitoring, this probably could have been avoided. After I got out of the hospital, I immediately changed physicians and finished my treatments with a new doctor. In this case, I probably should have acted even more quickly as it became apparent I could not receive adequate care from someone with twice the normal workload. I waited until it was safe to fire the doctor.

Firing your physician is a bold and frightening move, particularly if you are in the middle of treatment. Although many criteria can be appropriate grounds for a change, in my opinion, the overwhelming factor is your confidence that the physician is pursuing all options and has your best interests in mind. Over a ten-year period, I have switched physicians on four different occasions and have engaged a total of six oncologists, five surgeons, three radiologists, a neurologist and a physical therapist.

For those readers wondering how you fire a doctor, I would say that the approach depends on the situation and also on the type of insurance. Those who are covered under HMOs will probably need to go back through their medical organization and request a new physician, while those covered under PPOs (preferred provider option) or traditional indemnity plans are typically free to consult any physician. The most professional way to end a relationship is to write a letter notifying the old physician of the change and requesting that medical records be forwarded to the new physician.

While courteous, this is not absolutely necessary, as your new physician can always retrieve any necessary information.

## Finding a Doctor: Personal Referrals

In general, I strongly recommend personal referrals to physicians. Of course, you must keep in mind the source of the referral and how much credibility you give to the person's opinion. Since there are many factors at play here, it is wise to ask questions relating to the topics outlined earlier in this chapter. In my early selections of oncologists, I asked as many people as possible for recommendations and kept a tally of the names I was given. I chose the first doctor by tallying up the votes.

## Finding a Doctor: Physicians on the Insurance List:

One of my nurses commented that she is often surprised by patients who bring in lists of doctors who are approved by their HMO or PPO and ask her to tell them who they should go to. As a health professional, it amazed her that patients would risk sacrificing their health for a somewhat higher reimbursement from an unknown doctor, and would even change physicians for this reason. While many medical plans have a higher payout for doctors in the plan, almost all of them have a maximum out-of-pocket (usually in the $1,000-2,500 range) after which all approved costs are paid at 100 percent of what is "usual and customary." While costs may be an issue for some families struggling to maintain a reasonable lifestyle, I believe that to choose a physician based on whether or not they are on the list can be a disadvantageous practice. If finances are an issue, physicians will sometimes work with a patient to establish a payment plan.

## The Job of Being a Patient

Until confronted with an ongoing health problem, most people don't realize that being a patient is actually a *job* which requires a base of knowledge, a set of skills, organization, and ironically, a lot of *patience.*

The first thing you quickly learn is that being a patient is time-consuming. You must juggle multiple medical visits, second opinions, scans and other tests. With respect to complex illnesses which require many kinds of treatments, you often end up managing a diverse group of physicians and coordinating communication between them. I initially engaged a radiologist, a surgeon and a physical therapist. Soon after initial treatment, I acquired an oncologist (I now have two, one for daily operations and another for strategy consultation), a radiologist, a neurologist, and a special team for radio-surgery. The model of *general contractor* often comes to mind and I view myself as the head of a team that I must constantly manage, inform and, occasionally, even motivate.

Communication becomes a special problem when managing your medical records. Unfortunately, there is no true system for this in today's medical world. Individual treatment records are maintained by the local clinic or hospital department administering therapy. Since there is currently no centralized national database of medical records, reports and films must be faxed and/or physically transferred from one treatment facility to another. Requests for reports are often backlogged (it recently took me over three weeks to get a copy of an MRI report from my local hospital), and X-ray/CT/MRI scans often have to be hand carried from one doctor to another. I've gotten in the habit of maintaining my own set of reports which I take with me from specialist to specialist. I highly recommend this. In fact, for patients who have had a number of treatments over an extended period of time, it is very useful to maintain a written summary of your medical history that can be given to any new member of your team. I often surprise new physicians by giving them a write-up as part of my initial visit.

A second area of communication concerns getting quick feedback when new symptoms emerge or minor questions arise. Email can be a godsend with respect to efficient communication, especially when the patient has fears about new physical symptoms which may or may not be of clinical significance. Although email is widely used in the business world, physicians have been slow to embrace it, and computer technology in general. Once they have experienced its benefits, however, I have found they often will quickly adopt it as a much more efficient mode of communication. It also saves you from having to remain glued to your telephone for a return call. If possible, try to find a physician who uses email or is willing to consider it.

A third area of communication involves meetings with your physician. During appointments, communication tends to be rather abbreviated and, due to time constraints, the patient is often made to feel that asking too many questions should be avoided. Patients need to be prepared in advance to make the most of a five-to-ten minute appointment. I've gotten in the habit of compiling a list of questions and/or issues and telling my doctors up front that I have "five things to discuss," or four or three. This gives them a heads-up on roughly how much time I will need and avoids having them end the conversation prematurely. You should also be prepared to hand the doctor a written list to make sure all of the topics are covered.

## Key Insights: Choosing a Physician/Medical Team

- Recognize that historical bias plays a role in medicine and that many physicians gravitate toward tried and true methods.
- Ask for an initial consultation so that you can interview a potential new physician. Pay particular attention to whether they are open to a true partnership relationship.
- For chronic illnesses, physicians who are part of, or at least associated with, university research centers will often be the most up-to-date with respect to newer treatments.
- Look for flexibility and willingness to work with other physicians, attitudes which are very important when addressing difficult issues.

- Consider how aggressive the physician is with respect to treatment.
- Evaluate the clinical setting within which you will receive treatment and their attitude towards patient care.
- Look for a doctor with a positive attitude concerning your prognosis, one who will not give up when the going gets tough.
- Actively solicit personal referrals and note physicians who receive multiple recommendations.
- Don't be afraid to switch doctors if you are dissatisfied.
- Keep copies of major medical records at home.
- Realize that being a patient is like being a general contractor. It requires your active participation and management of the team and the process.

# Chapter 4

## Initial Decision Making: Process,

## Timeframe and Resources

After the initial diagnosis, there are many decisions to be made concerning treatment. This often must be done quickly, making it especially difficult. In non-emergency situations, I believe it is best to take a reasonable amount of time (as much as several weeks) to recover from initial shock, which may impair the ability to make rational decisions and learn about the disease.

### *Patient-to-Patient Counseling*

At the beginning, many patients find it useful to talk about their illness and suggested treatments with others who have been there, done that. Often, the patient's physicians can help provide links to others who are willing to talk to newly-diagnosed patients. In addition, many community service groups have established patient-to-patient or "buddy" systems and maintain an active database of volunteers. This can work well, especially if attention is paid to matching people based on age, personality and situation.

I spent considerable time talking with other breast cancer patients who were referred to me from a variety of sources, primarily personal friends and associates who had either been directly or indirectly affected by the illness. I was surprised by how knowledgeable many of these women were and how comforting it was to talk with someone who had actually survived the experience.

## Support Groups

An expanded version of patient-to-patient counseling may be found in support groups, which offer emotional support as well as some education in a group setting. While they may be more helpful in dealing with the effects of treatment or post-treatment issues, groups can also be useful on a drop-in basis for initial decision making. Meetings are often advertised through clinics, doctors and community service organizations. The more sophisticated organizations assemble groups according to demographics, such as age range, sex, individuals or couples. They can motivate patients to be more actively involved in seeking therapy and investigating best practices

## Private Counselors

There are also a number of private therapists and counselors who deal specifically with people facing life-threatening illnesses. They can often be found through support organizations, where many of them volunteer as group facilitators.

## Educational Services

Some medical clinics provide a nurse and/or patient education which can offer an overview of the illness and recommended treatments. Many communities and hospitals also maintain libraries/educational centers where patients can drop in and find help in researching their illness. In my own area in Northern California, I discovered these resources:

- Planetree Health Resources Centers and affiliates (located nationwide)

    o http://www.planetree.org/pat_welcome.html

- Community Breast Health Project in Palo Alto

    o http://www.cbhp.org

- Bay Area Breast Cancer Network in San Jose

    o http://www.babcn.org/

- The Ida and Joseph Friend Cancer Resource center at UCSF Comprehensive Cancer Center
- The Learning Center in Palo Alto

If you have access to the Internet, these resources can be found online, as a growing number create and maintain their own websites.

## Books

Books on almost all illnesses are readily available at local libraries and bookstores. Often, there will be a highly recommended book on a specific illness which becomes known as the bible for new patients. For breast cancer, this is undoubtedly *Dr. Susan Love's Breast Cancer Book*[5], which I have mentioned previously. For other cancers, patients should ask other patients as well as their physician for an initial recommendation.

It's also useful to buy a really good medical dictionary, because much of the terminology on reports will be unfamiliar and even downright scary. As with any field, the language is not nearly as intimidating once you understand it.

## Second Opinions

For any major health care decision, most people will want to obtain a second opinion. While many physicians will offer referrals, I believe it is best to find someone completely independent from your primary physician. Doctors often develop a small network upon which they rely to refer patients. If you remain within it, it

---

[5]    Love, Dr. Susan and Lindsey, Karen, *Dr. Susan Love's Breast Cancer Book,* Addison Wesley Publishers, 1995

is less likely that you will get a second opinion that differs considerably from the first.

I initially sought out someone who was well known in the research community at UCSF. Probably better known as a scientist than a clinician, his approach was largely based on a review of known literature as well as the statistics associated with outcomes of various treatments. My husband and I spent about an hour and a half in a consultation with him and walked away feeling we had a fairly good grasp of the range of possible outcomes. He took time to go through current as well as past research pertinent to my situation and even reviewed some international study results with us. While the visit with him did not change my initial treatment, it certainly made us feel that we were making a fully-informed decision and had a built a solid foundation for understanding future issues

## *Online Resources*

There are many health sites available online which offer a general overview of any illness, as well as more in-depth information on clinical trials and medical research.

If you are unfamiliar with the Internet or without a home computer, there are many local resources, including public libraries and educational centers associated with hospitals, that offer access and assistance. Friends and associates may also be willing to help with searches or offer a quick introduction to web surfing. New users can literally be using web browser software in a matter of minutes. Don't be intimidated by the technology: it offers truly incredible access to valuable information.

The Pew Internet and American Life Project (www.pewinternet.org) recently published a report listing the "Top Ten" most useful consumer health sites, as compiled by the Medical Library Association[6]:

---

[6]   Medical Library Association "Top Ten" Most Useful Consumer Health Web Sites, Pew Internet and American Life; http://www.pewinternet.org/reports/reports.asp?Report=59&Section=ReportLevel2&Field=Level2ID&ID=479

# The Top Ten list includes:

- Centers for Disease Control and Prevention (www.cdc.gov ), an agency of the Department of Health and Human Services
- Healthfinder (www.healthfinder.gov), a gateway consumer health information site
- HealthWeb:(www.healthweb.org), a site established by librarians and information professionals from academic medical institutions in the Midwest
- HIV InSite (www.hivinsite.ucsf.edu), a project of the University of California San Francisco AIDS Research Institute
- MayoClinic (www.mayoclinic.com), an online extension of the famed Mayo Clinic
- Medem (www.medem.com), a project of the leading medical societies in the U.S.
- MEDLINEplus (www.medlineplus.gov), a consumer-oriented site established by the National Library of Medicine, the world's largest medical library
- National Women's Health Information Center (www.4women.gov), a gateway to selected women's health information resources
- NOAH: New York Online Access to Health (www.noah-health.org), a collection of state, local and federal health resources for consumers
- Oncolink: A University of Pennsylvania Cancer Center Resource (www.oncolink.upenn.edu) the original and still leading site for information on various forms of cancer

Also recommended is:

- Medscape: (www.medscape.com), a general medical information site

## Putting It All Together

With so much information and support available, it can be daunting to select what's most useful. I believe it is wise to spend time educating yourself, first, by reading as much as you can, then speaking with others who have been through the experience and lastly, obtaining a second opinion or doing further online research. At that point, you can ask intelligent questions based on the knowledge that you have acquired. Although challenging, this can actually be done in two to three weeks, but it does take concentrated effort . . . and a little help from your friends.

Many people have also found it useful to ask their doctor a very basic question. "If it were your wife or someone you loved, what would *you* do?"

## Key Insights: Initial Decision Making

- Approach the educational process in steps, starting with getting a good grasp of the big picture before delving into details.
- Buy a good overview book as well as a comprehensive medical dictionary.
- Investigate educational facilities available in hospitals and your local community.
- Take a look at support groups to see if they would benefit you. Buddy systems can be especially useful.
- Get a second opinion from someone not associated with your doctor.
- Do an Internet search to find the best general sites for your condition. The American Library Association's "Top Ten" list is a good place to start.
- Realize that the learning process will be most intense for the first several weeks, but will last for the duration of your illness and, perhaps, beyond.

# Chapter 5

## Understanding the Medical Environment and

## How It Affects You

There are complex and diverse factors influencing how medicine is practiced in the U.S. today. While some of them are local or specific to the type of facility, others are a reflection of our ongoing national debate over access to medical care and the high costs associated with it. While I cannot address all of these issues in depth, there are certainly things that any new patient should keep in mind as they navigate our health care system.

## *Medical Infrastructure: Hospitals/Private Practices/ HMOs*

The type and quality of care that a patient receives often varies by the type of facility that is providing it. Staffing levels, government regulations, whether or not the institution incorporates teaching, reimbursement levels and even how physicians are managed, motivated, and compensated are all mitigating factors.

### *Hospitals/Nursing Care*

Most intensive medical care is delivered in hospital settings and is greatly dependent upon the quality of the nursing staff, since these are the professionals who have the most daily contact with patients. Recent legislation in California has mandated a minimum nurse-to-patient ratio for specific hospital care units, largely due to protests from nurses who are often overloaded and unable to deliver the quality of care they would like. One nurse I spoke with identified the practice of assigning nurses to "med surge" pools as a negative factor in patient care. Med surge pools are floating teams of nurses who may be deployed anywhere in a hospital depending on caseloads. While this may seem like a good idea, she was critical of the practice, noting that nurses, like doctors, develop specific areas of expertise and are best assigned to those units with which they are most comfortable and competent. For example, intensive care (ICU) nurses have different skills than oncology nurses.

## Teaching Hospitals

Teaching hospitals often incorporate interns into their daily patient care routines. While this is obviously beneficial to the students, it can be a detriment to the patient. It's difficult, for example, to have an intimate conversation with your physician with a group of interns watching. And I have on several occasions been subject to procedures performed by interns who were obviously getting on-the-job training. I had a bone marrow aspiration performed by an intern who was accompanied by an entourage of other students. She had obviously never done it before, seemed somewhat nervous and struggled to complete it. This caused extra anxiety as well as unnecessary discomfort for me. While it's hard to argue with the need for training, too often the interns are not adequately supervised. During another procedure, the resident had no idea of how to access a medi-port (a medical device implanted under the skin which gives ready access to the bloodstream), and was about to use the wrong needle. Had I not pointed out the problem, the mistake could have caused damage to the device, necessitating surgery to remove and replace it.

The point is that although one of the primary missions of a teaching hospital is to *teach*, this may at times compete with the delivery of the best possible patient care.

## Private Practice/Physician Autonomy

Autonomy is a powerful lure for private practice, in which doctors can create their own environment outside of the more structured hospital setting. As a result, one of my nurses commented that "doctors in private practice are more relaxed and seem more human with their patients." They also have more flexibility to prescribe specific drugs (hospitals often require doctors to use their own internal formularies) and to offer patients free samples which are provided by pharmaceutical companies.

Private practices also have the advantage of being focused on a specialty and often have on-site labs and other facilities which provide faster turn-around time—and more convenience—for their patients.

A new breed of private practice is beginning to emerge in some urban areas, prompted by physicians' desire to limit the quantity and maximize the quality of their interactions with patients. Based on a subscription model of service, they require patients to pay a retainer of several thousand dollars a year in return for a promise of immediate access and extended consultations: the guaranteed income permits a smaller patient load. Although this practice raises a host of issues with respect to insurance as well as the creation of a two-tier medical system, it will be interesting to see if this approach does, in fact, improve patient outcomes and overall satisfaction.

The downside of private practice is that physicians must work harder at maintaining contact with the research community. Many private physicians find it difficult enough to treat patients, deal with insurance companies and manage the administrative aspects of their practice. Attending research symposia and professional conferences may often be difficult. However, private practices seem to offer the best opportunity to develop a strong relationship with a physician, and the best doctors somehow find the time and energy to stay current with their specialties.

## HMO-Based Facilities

Patients who are covered by HMO plans should always be aware that cost containment is a major objective of these organizations. I discovered this quite accidentally after some particularly confusing encounters with my first oncologist. At the time, I was covered by the TakeCare HMO plan in California and receiving care at a local medical foundation which was largely HMO-based.

My first few sessions of chemotherapy left me suffering from nausea so intense that I could not work or even leave the house for extended periods. I asked my physician many times for more powerful anti-nausea drugs. She replied that she had given me everything available. I decided to do some research on my own and, after consulting with both my local pharmacist as well as a relative who was a physician, came up with the name of a new drug, odansetron hydrochloride (now marketed under the brand names of Zofran® and Kytril®). I went back to my oncologist and asked her about it.

Her answer was that it was still experimental and too expensive for me to use. At about $20 a day, I thought it would be well worth it if it could relieve my nausea. After a bit of badgering, she reluctantly gave me a prescription for Zofran®. It immediately reduced the nausea almost completely. During subsequent visits to this doctor, she almost invariably commented on the drug cost and tried to discourage my frequent use. I told her that it was so effective, I would pay for it myself if there was any problem with insurance coverage. Zofran® made the difference between being disabled and being able to work part-time.

I remained perplexed by this concern over the cost of the drug and the failure to be informed of its existence until I saw a documentary about TakeCare one evening on public television. Ironically, it focused on how this HMO's policies were being implemented at the clinic where my oncologist practiced, revealing that a fixed budget per disease was allotted to each patient. If doctors were able to manage costs within this amount, they would receive additional compensation.

I was horrified and astonished to find out that the quality of my care as well as my access to specific drugs had been manipulated by this system, and that my doctor, whom I trusted, might be profiting while I was suffering. When a couple of other incidents occurred with this facility, I changed to a private practice and converted to an indemnity insurance plan. I now ask much more pointed questions about *all* possible treatments.

## Managing Medicine Like a Business

A fundamental truth about medicine in the U.S is that it is a *business*. In fact, it has become one of the largest, currently consuming nearly 14 percent of our GNP and estimated to increase to 17 percent or $3 trillion within the decade. At this rate, medical care could consume up to one-third of the economy by mid-century.[7] Unfortunately, the economics of medicine are designed by the insurance companies, resulting in a system structured largely on reimbursement rates which typically run anywhere from 20 percent to 60 percent of the amount billed. This results in a conflict of interest for physicians, who are often forced to choose financial considerations over high-quality patient care.

At least one physician, Dr. Laura Esserman, who runs the Carol Frank Buck Breast Care Center at UCSF, would like to see medicine adopt other principals of business. With the benefit of M.D. and MBA degrees, her view of the actual "business" of medicine includes:

- Managing risks
- Minimizing morbidity
- Maximizing good outcomes
- Minimizing complications

While these may sound like the objectives of almost any business, it is interesting to consider medicine from this perspective. Most patients do not think of dealing with their illness in terms of risk. However, the uncertainty associated with many treatment regimens means that an evaluation of risk is a critical issue when making a decision.

---

[7]  Gleckman, Howard, *Welcome to the Health-Care Economy*, Business Week, Aug. 19-26, 2002

One relatively new thrust of research involving a combination of medicine and medical information technology, often called informatics, is developing models for understanding risk. Taking this a step further, a recent study[8] presented results of a physician-patient intervention designed to improve the quality of medical consultations between breast cancer patients and physicians, including treatment decisions, communication and overall satisfaction. The investigation looked at the benefit of having patients meet with a facilitator prior to consulting with their doctor to help them frame their questions and information needs. This was followed by a three-way session between the patient, physician, and facilitator, in which the facilitator was both an active participant and also a record-keeper. Patients with facilitators had significantly higher quality and satisfaction scores than those without. Presumably, they gained an increased understanding of treatment options, and risks and benefits associated with their specific cases. Still to be determined is the arguably more important question of whether or not the medical outcomes actually improved.

## Quality in Medicine

Business principles can be applied to the collection, measurement and dissemination of information concerning the quality and outcomes of medical care. A recent Bill Moyers special aired on PBS explored the issue of quality with respect to mammography and concluded that radiologist error was the most significant factor contributing to failure to detect cancer from mammograms. The program noted that there are no quality controls in radiology: a mammography facility can become certified merely by submitting films. Moyers went on to cite that even the best facilities have a detection rate of

---

8    Sepucha, K., Belkora, J., Tripahty, D., Esserman, L.: *Building Bridges Between Physicians and Patients: Results of a Pilot Study Examining New Tools for Collaborative Decision Making in Breast Cancer*. J. of clinical Oncology, Vol. 18, No 6 (March) 2000 pp 1230-1238

only 80 percent (meaning that 20 percent of cancers are *not* detected) and concluded that patients are playing a game of "radiologist roulette." The story ended with an anecdote about one place where the chief radiologist began firing radiologists with poor detection rates. This policy had a rapid and dramatic effect on improving the overall quality of the facility.

Dr. Esserman would like to see quality metrics applied to the measurement of outcomes for breast cancer patients. She cites an Institute of Medicine 1998 study which concludes that:

> "Serious and widespread quality problems exist throughout American Medicine . . . underuse, overuse, or misuse occurs in small and large communities alike, in all parts of the country, and with approximately equal frequency in managed care and fee-for-service systems of care. Quality of care is the problem, not managed care. Current efforts to improve will not succeed unless we undertake a major, systematic effort to overhaul how we deliver health care services, educate and train clinicians, and assess and improve quality."
>
> —Conclusions of the IOM Study, Chassin et al, JAMA 1998[9]

Dr. Esserman's vision incorporates a comprehensive database that tracks patient data and medical outcomes, with a major focus on quality of care. She foresees the day when outcomes and quality could be tracked and managed on a physician level, while acknowledging that access to and use of this information would involve a serious cultural change in the medical profession. There's

---

[9]   Chassin, M.R. and R.W. Galvin, *The urgent need to improve health care quality. Institute of Medicine National Roundtable on Health Care Quality.* Jama, 1998 **280**(11):p. 1000-5

a common saying in business: "If you can't measure it, you can't fix it." Despite the probable resistance from the medical community, better measurement of the quality of medical care probably represents one of the surest ways to improve it.

## *Manage Your Medical Affairs as You Would Any Other Business Interest*

Why is it important to start managing your own medical affairs the way you would any other business interest? First, realizing that the dynamics are the same allows for a degree of objectivity and takes a lot of the emotion out of the interaction. Second, maintaining a business perspective may provide an important set of tools for managing your own care. You must learn to use the same skills you've already developed in other areas of life, including the ability to do your own research, negotiate when appropriate and even charm others into seeing your point of view. They may come in handy when you're trying to persuade your physician to try something new and perhaps unproven. You will also learn to accept the fact that, like other professions, medicine has both strong and weak practitioners. The more you know about the system, the more successful you will be at sorting the good from the not-so-good and, ultimately, getting the best possible care.

The recognition that medicine is a business has resulted in important new legislation that provides additional protection to the consumer. A recently passed law allows patients to protest and even sue the managed healthcare industry's denial of certain treatments. Most businesses are rational. Knowledge of your rights as a consumer is a very important tool that you have in ensuring that you receive the best possible care.

## Key Insights: Understanding the Medical Environment

- Medicine is a business, with key objectives including risk management and maximization of outcomes.

- Differences exist in the level, quality, and convenience of care among hospitals, teaching hospitals, private practices, and HMO facilities.
- Patients are often unaware that physicians may have economic incentives to limit treatment options.
- Quality in health care is an ongoing debate in the medical profession and there is currently no systematic measurement of outcomes.
- Approaching your own medical care as you would any other business will help you to maximize the quality of what you receive.
- Keep up-to-date regarding laws that govern the quality of healthcare; it may mean access to life-saving or more comfortable treatment options.

# Chapter 6

## Ongoing Treatment

After enjoying nearly four years of cancer-free living following my initial treatment, a routine chest X-ray announced that I had suffered a massive recurrence in my lungs. I panicked, the same as I had with my initial diagnosis, only this time, I knew that it was far more serious. A relapse often means that the cancer has spread to other sites (a process known as metastasis) and has now become much more difficult to treat. My breast cancer had gone from something curable to the likelihood of becoming a chronic illness. A new set of strategies were required for treatment and decision-making, made somewhat easier by the fact I had an existing knowledge base about the illness and the timeframe was somewhat more generous. However, a relapse can be enormously stressful due to its implications for the long-term. Mine was no exception.

My experience has been that the health care system does a much better job of handling acute medical problems than dealing with ongoing ones, both on a physical as well as an emotional level. Acute problems can be dealt with fairly rapidly and usually have a clear outcome, either positive or negative. Chronic conditions create a lot of discomfort for both the physician and the patient as the treatments become long-term and the answers less certain.

The doctor/patient partnership model becomes particularly important here, as there are a variety of sources of information and experimental treatments available for metastatic cancer. It is likely that your physician will not be up-to-date on the wide range of experimental treatments, nor will he or she even have the time to research them. The patient often takes the lead in the search for new options and must be assertive about which ones to consider.

Although not yet emotionally prepared for this setback, I had already done some preliminary research on next steps. As any cancer patient will tell you, the fear of recurrence is always lingering in the back of their mind. My advance homework had indicated that a fairly radical treatment known as a stem cell transplant might hold the best possibility for a long-term remission—or even the remote possibility of a cure. At the time, this therapy was considered experimental and was officially monitored as a clinical trial by the government. It is a very expensive therapy and had recently been challenged by the insurance industry. Fortunately for me, all the cases had been decided in favor of patients and the industry was no longer denying benefits for treatment.

The stem cell transplant is a variant of a bone marrow transplant, in which the patient acts as his or her own donor of stem cells, the building blocks for many of the body's cells, including those of the immune system. This self-donation is known as an autologous transplant. As a cancer therapy, stem cells are removed from the blood and then stored cryogenically (frozen) while the patient is given massive doses of potent chemotherapy agents. Hopefully, the chemo kills most or all of the cancer cells, but it also destroys the immune system, leaving the patient vulnerable to infection.

My stem cells would be removed prior to treatment. I would be hospitalized for an extended period in a special stem cell ward and given what would be a near fatal dose of chemotherapy in an attempt to rid my body of all cancer cells. With my immune system destroyed, I would be temporarily supported with antibiotics and transfusions of both blood and platelets. Several days later, I would be rescued by a reintroduction of my own thawed stem cells. The reinfused cells would then regenerate my immune system over a period of about seven days. It sounded like a grueling procedure, which would require roughly a month of hospitalization followed by several additional months of recuperation.

Having decided that this was the most promising course to explore, I was sent by my oncologist to the transplant unit of a local hospital and medical school near my home for consultation. My husband and I spent about an hour discussing my case with the young doctor managing the program. She was decidedly negative about a positive outcome, citing the numerous areas of recurrence and noting that the procedure seemed to work best when confined to a small number of tumors or lesions. This argument didn't make a lot of sense either to me or my husband, since the procedure would either succeed or fail based on the underlying biological response of the individual malignant cells. The number of tumors seemed to us to be irrelevant. In fact, we suggested that my case might be a particularly *good* one since, although there were a large number of tumors, they were very small and would likely be readily penetrated by the chemotherapy.

We were surprised that the consulting physician disagreed and it became evident that she was negative about my being admitted as a patient. Slowly, I began to realize that this might not be my decision to make.

"Is this my decision or yours?" I asked.

"We would hope it is a mutual decision," she replied.

When asked for her recommendation, she began to talk about the progression of my illness and the possibility of using a hospice organization as my disease progressed to its final stages, which she obviously expected to happen in a relatively short timeframe. This effectively terminated the conversation. Dave and I left in a state of shock and disbelief that our access to this treatment had been blocked by the institution itself. It didn't occur to us that another place and other physicians might look at the same data and reach very different conclusions.

Shortly after that I went back on chemotherapy, using a regimen that I had discovered through visiting a doctor in Southern California who had been recommended by a relative in the medical profession. It required alternating two different drugs, which were administered continuously over the course of a week through use of a mobile pump. This was, at the time, an aggressive and unusual approach. I made the connection between this physician and my principal oncologist, insisting that we try this. Within a few weeks, the new technique was already starting to show some dramatic results in reducing the size and number of lesions in my lungs.

Emboldened by success, Dave and I did more research and traveled to another well-known medical institution fifty miles away that also specialized in stem cell transplants for breast cancer. We repeated the same interview process without letting anyone know we had already been turned down by another hospital. This time, the consulting physician was quite positive, with the principal investigator urging me to undergo the procedure.

"I wouldn't even think about not doing this," he said. "We can absolutely help you."

I quizzed him about the effectiveness of the therapy, given the number of small tumors involved, and he confirmed our initial thoughts, noting that the number was independent of the effectiveness of the therapy. "If it works on one tumor," he said, "it is likely to work on all of them." We decided to keep to ourselves the fact that this second opinion was diametrically opposite the first.

When I indicated that I would like to go ahead with the transplant, he called in several other team members to talk to me. They reviewed the treatment plan, timetable and possible complications and then one of the team members said he had just one question.

"We are curious as to why you selected this hospital when there is another institution that is so much closer to you. Why don't you get your treatment closer to home?"

My husband and I looked at each other, gulped and then went ahead and told them what had happened. The room was silent when we were finished. Eventually one of the doctors mumbled, "Well, perhaps they might have come to a different conclusion if they had seen the response you are getting to the therapy you are on right now." Despite this rather meek attempt to defend their colleagues, it was clear that they were shocked that I had been turned down.

As I grew more knowledgeable about clinical trials and results, I became aware that, for experimental or new treatments, patients are sometimes selected based on the principal investigator's evaluation or, perhaps, intuition, of how likely they are to benefit from the therapy and become a favorable statistic for the study. Since I had not yet resumed chemotherapy and seen an immediate benefit, the first facility I visited had no evidence that a transplant would be beneficial, but the second facility did. While I don't believe this is a common issue with respect to trials, the politics of medicine seemed to intrude in my case.

I underwent the transplant and, following a challenging recovery, gained another thirteen months of cancer-free life before new problems emerged. Although the allure of a cure had seemed within reach, it did not materialize. As with many of the newer medical treatments, I had taken a calculated gamble and gone through a very tough procedure. Already in remission prior to the beginning of the stem cell treatment, I now believe it possible that the extended remission would have happened anyway. In fact, recent studies have shown that there appears to be little long-term benefit from stem cell transplants for breast cancer and they are now being done less frequently. Nevertheless, I had a thirteen-month remission. This still appears to be a reasonable outcome, even allowing for the discomfort. The lesson here is understanding that experimental treatments, even promising ones, don't always have good long-term benefits. But at the end of the day, this one kept me alive long enough to take advantage of Herceptin®, which provided another two-year remission.

## Clinical Trials

Clinical trials can be a lifeline for those who have failed conventional therapy. The experimental nature of the stem cell procedure stimulated my interest in the growing number of emerging cancer treatments and the trials that are used to evaluate their safety and efficacy.

Basically human experiments with newly proposed drug therapies which have proven to be beneficial in animal studies, there are three levels of clinical trials known as Phase I, Phase II, and Phase III. They are conducted according to procedures specified by the FDA and investigators must get government approval before proceeding with tests on human volunteers. A drug which successfully passes all three levels will be approved for a specific medical use by the FDA.

Phase I trials are set up to test for the overall safety of a proposed drug. The number of patients admitted is typically very small, numbering in the dozens.

Phase II trials test for efficacy of the drug on a larger selection of patients, typically numbering in the hundreds. These may or may not include a control group (i.e., patients receiving some alternative therapy or a placebo, but not the active agent under investigation). This phase can last as long as a couple of years.

Success will lead to a Phase III trial, which can involve thousands of patients and is meant to test for the effectiveness on a specific population which may be helped by the therapy. It is expensive to run because of the number of people involved and its duration: a Phase III trial is often conducted over a number of sites across the country and may last up to five years. You can begin to see why new drugs and new treatments can be so expensive and take so long to reach the market.

The media is often quick to pick up on early clinical trial results, particularly when a new drug can be life-saving for a particular patient population. Unfortunately, many drugs which appear promising in animal tests fail to produce adequate benefits in people and fall out of the process during Phase I and II trials. About 80 percent of drugs that make it to Phase III are ultimately approved.[10] Ironically, the lack of new patients for clinical trials is one of the key impediments to the more rapid deployment of new therapies: it is estimated that only about five percent of all cancer patients enroll in clinical trials. Awareness is a key issue, with almost 85 percent of patients unaware of existing trials. Other factors include

---

[10] Lemonick, Michael D. and Goldstein, Andrew, *At Your Own Risk,* Time Magazine, April 22, 2002

clinical physicians' lack of knowledge, difficulty associated with accessing trial information and even the primary physician's fear of losing patients to a trial doctor.

*Physician Awareness*

Physicians are often woefully ignorant of clinical trials, partly because their patient load absorbs the majority of their free time while dealing with insurance companies, staff and the occasional professional conference consumes the balance. In addition, there is no good mechanism for keeping them informed, with the recruitment of new patients often done quite casually through existing networks of physicians already connected to a research institution and/or pharmaceutical company.

With doctors often acting as gatekeepers, it is not surprising that more patients do not enroll. New avenues for physician outreach may be critical to recruiting more patients: the NCI is currently focused on this.

*Patient Access to Trial Information*

The burden of researching trials and making contact with investigators primarily falls upon the patient. While patients can be successful in recruiting their doctors to contact trial coordinators on their behalf, identification of the trial of interest is often done by the patient, particularly if the trial site is not local. This demands an unusual level of proactive involvement.

Currently, research can be done largely over the Internet with data made available by the National Cancer Institute, as well as a few additional websites.

*1) PDQ Sponsored by the National Cancer Institute*

The National Cancer Institute (NCI) offers general information on cancer clinical trials and how they are performed as well as a search screen which can be used to search a database (known as the

PDQ database) of over four thousand cancer clinical trials. It is currently considered the premier site for cancer trials in the U.S.

http://www.cancer.gov/cancer_information/
http://www.cancer.gov/clinical_trials/
http://www.cancer.gov/search/clinical_trials/

This database has been updated a number of times over the past several years and now exists in both patient-friendly and more technically-oriented—for physician—formats. Searches can be refined to select trials based on a number of criteria:

- Stage of the cancer
- Geographical preference
- Type of treatment
- Trial phase (I, II or III)
- Trial sponsor

## 2) *ClinicalTrials.gov Sponsored by the NIH and NLM*

Another important resource is sponsored by the National Institute of Health and developed by the National Library of Medicine at www.clinicaltrials.gov. It offers the most comprehensive central listing of clinical studies sponsored by the NIH, other federal agencies, the pharmaceutical industry and nonprofit organizations in the U.S. The PDQ database is included, but the site also covers a wide range of illnesses beyond cancer.

## 3) *Private Sector Clinical Trials Listing Service*

A number of private trial listing services have also popped up to serve a growing variety of illnesses. Some of them will automatically notify the patient when a new trial of interest is posted. While the business model for most of these services is still developing, many rely heavily on the recruitment of patients for trials with a fee paid by the sponsoring/listing organization (usually a pharmaceutical company).

CenterWatch (http://www.centerwatch.com) is one such commercial site that lists 41,000 industry and government sponsored clinical trials. It offers the patient notification via email as new trials of interest are posted to the site. This is strictly an online listing with no active matching of patients to specific trials.

Emerging Med is another recently established site which does try to match patients to existing trials (http://www.emergingmed.com). It collects information relevant to the patient's current status and provides a match against trials that are posted to or otherwise referenced by their database. As a commercial for-profit venture, it receives payment from pharmaceutical companies for each patient enrolled.

It is important for patients to keep in mind that comprehensive databases with all known trials for a given illness do not exist at this time. The National Cancer Institute, for instance, primarily posts trials that have received NCI funding. While these include many important studies, there are others at private research institutes and pharmaceutical companies. Patients should check all of the sources listed above, as well as investigate trials that may be available through local research universities and often listed on the university's own web sites.

*Medical News:*

Late-breaking news on trials and drugs which seem promising can also be found by using news search engines including:

- PR News Wire

  o   http://www.prnewswire.com/news/

- Eureka Alert!

  o   http://www.eurekalert.org

- Biospace

    o http://www.biospace.com/news.cfm

- Business Wire Search

    o http://www.businesswire.com/

- Breast Cancer News
    o http://www.breastcancer.net
    o (subscription service available for a nominal fee—covers latest news bulletins on breast cancer research. Updated daily.)

*Contact with Trial Coordinators*

Following identification of a trial of interest, a patient must either directly or indirectly (i.e., through their physician) contact the trial coordinator to determine eligibility. Trials are conducted on a very specific patient population, which requires that patients meet a pre-determined set of medical requirements. These criteria serve to define a grouping of patients who are more or less similar, an experimental technique designed to reduce variability in the outcomes. They may be fairly complex, requiring that the patient meet multiple conditions in terms of prior treatments, age and current medical status.

In addition, many, although not all, of the studies are *randomized* and *double-blind*, meaning that patients may be assigned to either the active or a control group for statistical comparison. Double-blind indicates that neither the patient nor the investigator know which assignment has been made. Control groups typically receive some type of therapy, but do not receive the active agent being tested.

Occasionally, patients can obtain access to a drug outside of a trial based on a practice known as compassionate use. This is determined by the specifics of an individual case, the stage of drug testing and company policy. Compassionate use requests should be made directly to the pharmaceutical company that manufactures the drug or to the trial sponsor. Persistence can make a difference! A notable example is the early access to Herceptin® which was established by Genentech in response to pressure from the breast cancer community. When encouraging results from trials prompted demand for the drug prior to final approval by the FDA, anxious patients and breast cancer advocates lobbied both the company and the media for access to the limited supplies. Their efforts resulted in a quarterly lottery system which provided Herceptin® to qualified patients on a compassionate use basis.

*Enrollment and Treatment*

Since treatment through clinical trials is administered only at the trial sites involved in the investigation, the patient must often travel. The frequency of travel and type of therapy varies widely, depending on the trial. Prior to my second recurrence, I enrolled in a trial for a cancer vaccine being conducted at the University of Washington. I discovered it by doing research on the PDQ database and contacted the researcher directly in Seattle. Although my initial contact indicated that I was indeed eligible, I was subsequently informed that the trial had been filled and was closed to new patients.

Although discouraged, I continued to maintain contact with the coordinator and eventually gained acceptance through sheer persistence. The study involved a series of six vaccinations: the first vaccination required allergy testing over a twenty-four-hour period and necessitated an overnight stay. With subsequent appointments requiring only a few hours, I found it an easy day trip up and back from the San Francisco Bay Area. I was impressed with the care I received and the level of interaction with the nurses and researchers. Unfortunately, I had to drop out of the study after the fourth visit due to a recurrence which required that I immediately begin active treatment with Herceptin®. Since the vaccine was designed to stimulate a

natural immune response similar to the artificial one that
Herceptin® provides, this treatment invalidated my continuing
participation. Nevertheless, it was a positive experience and I
do not regret the time and effort.

With clinical trials, it is typical for the patient to pay for her
own travel arrangements while actual therapy and any associated
medical costs are covered by the research facility. For patients with
restricted budgets, travel can sometimes be arranged through a
charitable organization known as the Corporate Angel Network
(CAN). This organization provides free air transportation for cancer
patients using the empty seats on corporate jets. More information
can be found at: http://www.corpangelnetwork.org/

Enrollment in any trial involves risks and requires the patient
to sign a number of liability releases. However, the medical facility/
hospital associated with the study typically agrees to provide any
medical treatment necessary as a result of side effects. It is
important that patients have a clear understanding of this aspect
since insurance does not always cover costs associated with clinical
trials.

A rather unpleasant exception to this occurred during my
investigation of a trial being conducted at Memorial Sloan-Kettering
Cancer Center in New York. Having flown across the country to
discuss my possible participation, I was surprised to be given a
form indicating I would be charged for all office visits and blood
tests associated with the study. Upon my return home, I was
shocked to receive a bill for $500 for the initial interview with the
investigator. Since this had not been discussed in advance and was
clearly out of the ordinary, I refused to pay it. After many phone
calls and much negotiation, the fee was dropped.

This experience, however, emphasizes the need for patients to
understand both what they are getting involved with as well as
what is considered customary and usual for clinical trials. I consider
this second encounter to be an anomaly and I continue to be
impressed by the quality of care and attention paid to trial
participants. But patients should ask *all* the hard questions before
committing to *any* trial.

*The Need for a National Registry*

When first diagnosed, I became aware of, and later good friends with, a co-worker who had lymphoma. I did quite a bit of research for her and was constantly encouraging her to consider clinical trials. One conversation we had made a particularly deep impression on me.

"I can't believe," she said, "that you will just call anyone, anywhere in the country, and talk to them about your illness and their research. I just can't do that."

Despite the intense discussion that followed, she continued to be reluctant to follow-up and unfortunately, died despite the availability of an experimental treatment that was known to have up to a 40 percent cure rate. I have often considered the tragedy of shyness actually preventing access to a potentially life-saving option.

Such reluctance is understandable among patients who are overwhelmed by the illness itself and are then called upon to do their own research and outreach. I have advocated and begun work with two other women to develop a system that is "patient-centric" as opposed to "research-centric." The dream for this new model is to allow breast cancer patients to enter their specific medical history into an online registry, which could then be made available to interested researchers on a secure basis. Patients matched to specific trials would be privately notified and invited to contact a trial coordinator for possible enrollment. The service would be strictly not-for-profit to minimize any potential conflicts associated with payments received for patient participation. While it is still in development, our hope is that it will both accelerate participation in trials as well as relieve patients of one more burden of their illness. A national registry for all patients interested in clinical trials, irrespective of their illness, is the ultimate goal. An early version of this system is now being tested.

# Medical Research, Conferences/Seminars/Scientific Articles

Regular research conferences and seminars exist for almost every major illness: they vary from large annual national conferences to seminars and smaller focused meetings held at universities and major medical centers. An excellent resource for information is Medscape (www.Medscape.com), a commercial site recently acquired by WebMD. It includes a significant searchable database of conference information and reporting. In the cancer world, the major U.S. conference is ASCO (American Society of Clinical Oncologists), held annually in May. Also of importance is the San Antonio Breast Cancer Symposium in San Antonio, Texas.

Smaller gatherings, although not as well advertised, can usually be found by contacting local medical schools or searching the university's website. I recently attended two excellent seminars held at Stanford University on cutting-edge cancer topics. The first was on the developing field of Angiogenesis, a current hot topic in cancer research. It featured Dr. Judah Folkman, who has pioneered this field for more than a decade. At smaller conferences, patients (if they are not shy!) can often make direct contact with the speakers and even get advice. The second seminar covered the many uses of stem cells, including their use in transplants for cancer patients. This gave me some insight as to why my stem cell transplant had failed to provide the elusive cure as well as what might be done to improve effectiveness.

Patients who become actively involved in the research world, and have the interest and skills, are occasionally given an opportunity to speak at conferences. If this is your cup of tea, it can be an excellent way to broaden your network of contacts and often encourages researchers to approach you directly. Like most things in life, who you know can provide an important edge in the fight.

One of the premier resources for doing detailed scientific research is at the National Library of Medicine's online web site which represents the world's largest biomedical library at: www.nlm.nih.gov. It also has a link to Medline/Pub Med, which includes online references and abstracts to over 4,300 scientific journals and can be accessed directly at: www.ncbi.nlm.nih.gov/entrez/query.fcgi

Of course, detailed medical research can be challenging and frustrating if you do not have a background in biology or medicine.

A good medical dictionary will go a long way towards helping decipher the sometimes intimidating vocabulary. Despite my willingness to tackle this, I found that reading abstracts and published articles was not the most effective way of discovering new therapies. Most research reported in journals will be years away from being translated into clinical practice. Better sources are public television specials on cutting edge therapies, online medical news sites, community service groups focused on offering support and education to patients and even the popular press. At a minimum, these more informal sources can serve to pinpoint promising new agents or procedures which then can be followed via the more formal technical information sources.

## Support Groups

Support groups exist for nearly all illnesses and serve to draw together a group of people who are experiencing a similar life challenge. They may be organized by hospital and clinic educational programs or more commonly by outside community service groups. They are often advertised on bulletin boards in doctor's offices, at medical clinics, in the community service sections of local newspapers and on the Internet.

Usually loosely organized, support groups often meet on a weekly basis and are typically run by volunteers who may have a background in psychology and/or group counseling. They are frequently categorized according to patient population and stage of disease. For cancer patients, newly diagnosed patients are often organized separately from those dealing with a recurrent or chronic condition. Sometimes they are also categorized based on life stage, such as young mothers or married couples. Different populations have different concerns and may, in fact, be at odds with each other (as in the case of groups dealing with recurrent illness).

Whether or not a support group works for any individual person really depends on what the patient is looking for as well as the group's dynamics. In newly diagnosed situations, they are almost always helpful for education and the comfort that come with sharing a common experience. On an ongoing basis, groups can be a source of support, but you must be careful to select one that has a balanced emotional tempo. There were several members of an early group I joined who had particularly negative outlooks and served to depress everyone rather than provide inspiration and encouragement. In fact, one of the members invited me to attend a funeral service designed to mourn her surgery site. This didn't work for me. At the other extreme, several years later one of my physicians connected me to a patient needing support. Joanne and I became friends and often partner on breast cancer projects. We share an interest in focusing on a cure and in state-of-the-art research. She has, in fact, become even more diligent than I am in keeping up-to-date on new developments and often sends news flying my way via email. These include a variety of remedies, both medical as well as holistic. Because of her, I have now added daily doses of green tea, soy milk and flax seed to my regimen. I found one-on-one support to work much better for me, but each patient needs to experiment with these groups and find their own groove.

There is evidence that support groups can improve both the quality as well as quantity of life in certain situations. Studies conducted by Dr. David Spiegel at Stanford University, first published in 1989, demonstrated that patients with metastatic breast cancer who participate in support groups tend to live longer than those who do not.[11] This finding has been controversial and Spiegel himself admits it was unexpected. He is currently conducting a new study designed to validate his earlier findings. One possible interpretation of his research would be that the results are due to an experimental design error known as selection bias. More aggressive patients tend to enroll in these groups and these are the ones who are actively seeking help, looking for new therapies

---

[11]   Spiegel, D, Bloom, Jr, Kraemer HC and Gottheil E (1989) *Effect of psychosocial treatment of survival of patients with metastatic breast cancer.* The Lancet, 888-891.

and in control of their care. Of course, they are exactly the kind of patients that this book hopes to encourage!

## *Summary of Online Resources:*

*For clinical trials:*

- PDQ/National Cancer Institute
  http://www.cancer.gov/cancer_information/
  http://www.cancer.gov/clinical_trials/
  http:// www.cancer.gov/search/clinical_trials/
- ClinicalTrials.gov sponsored by the NIH and NLM
  http://clinicaltrials.gov
- CenterWatch
  http://www.centerwatch.com/
- EmergingMed www.emergingmed.com

*For health related news (search on related illness):*

- PR News Wire
  www.prnewswire.com/news/
- Eureka Alert!
  http://www.eurekalert.org
- Biospace
  www.biospace.com/news/cfm
- Business Wire Search
  www.businesswire.com
- Breast Cancer News
  www.breastcancer.net

*Medical research and medical conferences:*

- Medscape (now part of WebMD): resource for public medical conferences
  www.medscape.com

- National Library of Medicine: (world's largest biomedical library)
  www.nlm.nih.gov/
- Medline/PubMed sponsored by the NLM and offering online abstracts and detailed scientific journal articles
  www.ncbi.nlm.nih.gov/entrez/query.fcgi

## Key Insights: Ongoing Treatment

- Investigate clinical trials available for your illness using the Internet.
- Learn about medical conferences pertinent to your situation and consider attending them.
- Contact your nearest medical school/university to see if there are any seminars on research pertaining to your illness.
- The Internet has become as astounding resource for medical information. If you have a computer and service provider, use them. If not, find Internet access any way you can and learn to use what may be a lifesaving tool.
- Consider joining a support group or local community group that provides services and information to patients.
- Work at expanding your network to include people most knowledgeable about your illness.

# Chapter 7

## Emerging Therapies: The Road Ahead

Although this is not a medical reference, I believe it is useful to offer readers some current information about new and emerging therapies, particularly those which proved so helpful to me personally. This chapter will give a brief but current overview of some selected new therapies: noninvasive radiosurgery, minimally invasive radio-frequency ablation, monoclonal antibodies and anti-angiogenesis. The first two techniques involve processes which are effective in actively killing localized tumors at specific locations in the body. The second two therapies focus on areas of research which use biological approaches to systemically kill tumor cells all over the body. The biological approaches, which are targeted to specific characteristics of cancer cells, appear to hold the most promise for the future control of cancer, particularly that which has metastasized to other parts of the body.

## *Noninvasive/ Stereotactic Radiosurgery*

In contrast to traditional radiation therapy, which exposes a relatively large area of the body to ionizing or cell-killing radiation, stereotactic radiotherapy is a non-invasive form of radiation that is targeted specifically to a tumor site. This specificity spares surrounding tissue from the damaging effects of radiation. It is available in two flavors: an older technology known as the Gamma Knife and a newer, more comfortable version marketed under the name CyberKnife®. Following my treatment, I was so enamored with its possibilities that I conducted interviews with both the staff who administered it and the company that developed it. Based on these interviews, I wrote the following article which was published in a local breast cancer newsletter.

## Radiosurgery—the New Frontier
### By Joan E. Schreiner

On June 18th, I underwent CyberKnife® radiosurgery at Stanford for the treatment of two metastatic brain lesions. This surgery did not require any anesthesia, no incisions were made, no pain was involved and recovery was limited to a long afternoon nap. It was by far the easiest treatment for breast cancer that I've received in an 8-year-long battle.

Stanford's CyberKnife® is currently one of only five next-generation radio surgery devices in the U.S. produced by a local company, Accuray. The device produces very precise doses of focused radiation enabling a surgeon to use radiation as a substitute for a knife. Currently in use for brain and cervical spinal lesions, the radiation can be targeted to 1mm accuracy and delivered in a single treatment session.

Radiosurgery differs from conventional radiation therapy in that it utilizes an intense dose of targeted radiation to destroy a tumor in a single session, as opposed to multiple treatments. In addition, the ability to precisely target a tumor spares the surrounding tissue the radiation dose that would be received from the less focused approach of radiating an entire treatment field.

The CyberKnife® is the successor to an older technology called the gamma knife, which is also capable of delivering focused radiation. The gamma knife utilizes a stereotactic frame system to facilitate targeting, which requires patients to wear a head-mounted metal frame system for stabilization. This system requires a very firm attachment to the head through the use of temporary screws. The "frameless" CyberKnife® offers an obvious advantage in terms of patient comfort. In addition, CyberKnife®'s image guidance system and real-time target adjustment offers the potential to treat tumors in areas of the body (such as the lungs) which may be in motion during treatment.

My treatment involved a three-step outpatient procedure. The process began with construction of a face mask which is used as a head stabilization device during treatment. This involves a process that is no more daunting than receiving a facial, during which a plastic mold was made of my face and head. This mask is then utilized during a high resolution CT scan which produces the data needed for treatment planning, as well as during the treatment itself. I was able to leave the hospital after completing this initial set-up, which took only about two hours.

The imaging data is then utilized by the "surgeon" to construct a treatment plan, which involves identifying the exact size, shape and location of the tumor to be treated, as well as the number, intensity and direction of the radiation beams that will be directed at the target.

I returned two days later for the actual treatment. I had not yet seen the CyberKnife® in action, but got a quick preview when I observed another patient being treated.

The actual device consists of a robotic arm, which is capable of moving completely around the patient at varying angles. The arm is attached to a small linear accelerator which produces the radiation. The patient wears the facial mask during treatment as a head stabilization device; however, two sensors located on either side of the head constantly collect x-ray images which are compared to the original CT scan. Prior to each dose of radiation, the exact head positioning is computed and the appropriate adjustment is made to the robotic arm to compensate for any head movement. This entire process is monitored on an image guidance system driven by a high-powered Silicon Graphics Octane computer system. Having worked for SGI for seven years, I was particularly proud of this application of the company's technology and grateful to be a beneficiary of it.

Perhaps the most interesting part of the radiation delivery is the actual dose concentration. While each beam of radiation penetrates all the way through the treatment path, a single beam consists of a sub-therapeutic dose. It is only at the site of the tumor target that the cumulative dose is received.

When it was my turn to receive the treatment, I hopped up onto a narrow bed similar to a CT platform. The mask was applied and everyone left the room. I was alone with the CyberKnife®, while my surgical team was actually monitoring the robotic delivery in a separate observation room. The only sounds were a mild whirring from the robotic arm as well as some mechanical noises from the x-ray machines. I felt absolutely nothing during the actual treatment delivery. Each lesion took about an hour to treat, with a brief break in between.

At the end of the session, I was greeted by Dr. David Martin, who had prepared my treatment plan and who happily exclaimed "those pesky tumors are gone!" He also asked me to smile when I walked past the waiting room since I would be observed by the next set of patients. On my way out I looked around the room, turned both thumbs up and said "Don't worry, it was a piece of cake." You could feel the tension in the room dissolve as everyone laughed and thanked me. Many thanks to my treatment team at Stanford which included Dr. Steven Chang, Dr. David Martin, Larry Jang, Jennie Hai, and Tony Ho.

Although Stanford has primarily focused on treatment of brain and spinal cord lesions, which are approved uses of the CyberKnife®, they have recently expanded this therapy to include treatment of lung lesions. It is also exciting to note that recently an upgrade of the CyberKnife® has received government approval for treatment of tumors anywhere in the body. It is encouraging to envision the day when "pesky tumors" anywhere in the body can be treated by a procedure that is so comfortable and easy for the patient.

More information about Accuray can be found at the company's website www.accuray.com, or by contacting:

**Accuray Incorporated**
Wendy Wifler, Director of Marketing and Placement Services
570 Del Rey Ave.
Sunnyvale, CA 94085
Tel: (408) 522-3740 x286; Fax: (408) 830-0481
Email: info@accuray.com

Current CyberKnife® installations in the U.S. include the following:

**Shadyside Hospital**
5230 Centre Avenue
Pittsburgh, PA 15232
(412) 623-6720 or 623-2121
UPMC Shadyside Hospital
5230 Centre Avenue
Pittsburgh, PA 15232
http://www.neurosurgery.pitt.edu/microneurosurgery/cyberknife.html

**University of Texas**
**Southwestern Medical Center**
5323 Harry Hines Blvd.
Dallas, TX 75390-9122
(214) 648-7684 (Referrals)
http://www2.utsouthwestern.edu/radiationoncology/
cyberknife.htm

**CyberKnife at Newport Diagnostic Center**
1605 Avocado Avenue
Newport Beach, CA 92660
(949) 760-3024 or (800) 605-5170
http://www.newportdiagnosticcenter.com/cyberknife.html

**Cleveland Clinic Cancer Center**
9500 Euclid Avenue, T28
Cleveland, OH 44195
(216) 445-6645
http://www.clevelandclinic.org/radonc/corcam/default.htm
Email: cyberknife@radonc.ccf.org

**Georgetown University**
3800 Reservoir Road NW
Washington, DC 20007
(202) 784-2000

http://www.georgetownuniversityhospital.org/body.cfm?id=451
EMail: info@hospital.org

**USC/Norris Comprehensive Cancer Center and Hospital**
1441 Eastlake Avenue
Los Angeles, CA 90033-0804
(800) USC-CARE
http://www.uscnorris.com/services/cyberknife/information.htm

**UCSF Medical Center**
505 Parnassus Avenue
San Francisco, CA 94122
(415) 353-8900
  (Cyberknife non-spine radiosurgery)
(415) 353-2383
  (Cyberknife spine radiosurgery)

**Rocky Mountain CyberKnife Center**
**Boulder Community Hospital**
905 Alpine Avenue
Boulder, CO 80301
Ph: (303) 938-5353
http://www.boulderneuro.com/site/index.html

**Stanford University Medical Center**
300 Pasteur Drive
Stanford, CA 94305
Neurosurgery: (650) 723-5573
www.stanford.edu/group/neuorology/
PR: Ruthann Richter (650) 725-8047

Physician contacts at these facilities as well as a list of international
facilities are available on the company's website at:

  http://www.accuray.com/contact/
  site_locations.htm

## Radiofrequency Ablation for Liver Tumors

Radiofrequency ablation (also known as RF ablation) has been used as a therapy to treat liver tumors, both primary and metastatic. Since liver metastasis is so common in breast cancer, it is an important tool in the arsenal of treatments for advanced disease.

The technique relies on the ability of radiofrequency (or RF) energy delivered by an electrode to heat and destroy (ablate) localized tumor cells. Although not a cure for widespread cancer, it can be used to successfully treat single or even multiple solid tumors in the liver and, potentially, other organs. The liver is well suited to this technique since its extensive blood supply acts to dissipate heat very quickly, thus resulting in minimal damage to tissue outside the ablation zone. As one of the most regenerative organs in the body, the liver will also replace damaged portions of itself over time.

As a laparoscopic procedure, RF is considered to be minimally invasive. It usually involves two to three small abdominal incisions for placement of a video camera, a laparoscopic ultrasound device and the ablation needle or electrode. The combination of video and ultrasound allows the surgeon to evaluate the location of the tumor and place the ablation needle in the appropriate spot. The needle is heated using a radio-frequency generator to a temperature of approximately 113°F for fifteen minutes to complete the ablation. As the tissue is heated, dissolved gases form micro-bubbles which can be monitored by ultrasound to confirm that the treated cells have been destroyed. The needle can then be moved to a new position if multiple ablations are required (as in the case of a large tumor or with multiple tumors).

Having discovered in one of my routine scans that a previously detected but quiescent liver tumor had begun to grow alarmingly, I underwent this procedure which required only an overnight stay in the hospital. The primary complication from the surgery was abdominal discomfort from nitrogen gas which is used to pump up the abdomen so the surgeon is able to better visualize and separate the internal organs. Unfortunately, the gas does not dissipate very quickly and can be fairly uncomfortable for a period of time lasting days or even weeks. The procedure has worked quite well (92 percent success rate), on tumors up to 5cm and has achieved an 88 percent success rate with larger tumors. Because of the size of my lesion, we were unable to ablate all of it in the first operation, so I required a second procedure five months later to clear the residual tumor. I am happy to report that it appears to have been a success.

Patients are monitored with follow-up CT scans at three-month intervals, during which the area ablated gradually liquefies and is reabsorbed by the body. Re-treatment is possible in the event of a recurrence.

Eligibility for treatment with RF ablation depends on the number of lesions, overall size and the proximity to major blood vessels (which may limit the effectiveness of the treatment due to their cooling effect as heat is applied). Pioneering work in this area has been done at the University of California, San Francisco, although treatment is also available at other facilities in the U.S. A more extensive write-up is available on the UCSF website at: http://rfa.ucsf.edu.

General information about the RF ablation device is available from the manufacturer, Rita Medical Systems, located in Mountain View, California. Their website also includes a link to a directory of physicians across the country using this technique: http://www.ritamedical.com/index.htm

## Monoclonal Antibodies

The human body recognizes the presence of foreign invaders including disease-causing bacteria, viruses and other infectious agents as antigens. Antibodies are produced by the immune system as a normal reaction to the presence of an antigen; they can bind to a specific intruder and block its activity. They have some very useful characteristics, including their ability to confer long-term resistance to an antigen, a response known as immunization (the basic principle behind all vaccines), as well as their extreme specificity for targeting a particular molecule. Antibodies can kill and often control diseases by destroying infected cells or, in the case of bacteria, the invading cells themselves.

The ability of antibodies to attack specific disease agents has generated intense interest among researchers working on human therapies that target cancer cells. The presence of either unique molecules on the surface of certain cancer cells or molecules over-expressed by cancer cells makes them susceptible to treatment with artificial antibodies coupled with chemotherapy that can be targeted for delivery to a malignant cell.

Traditionally, production of antibodies has relied on injecting laboratory animals, typically mice, with the antigen of interest and then collecting the antibodies produced by the animal. This method has limitations due to impurities in the many different cell lines in the animal (known as polyclonal) as well as low yields of useful product. Monoclonal antibody technology was developed as a way to provide large amounts of pure antibodies. The technique involves a complicated process which requires fusion of a mammalian cell line with a tumor cell that can replicate endlessly. This results in a pure cell line—monoclonal—known as a hybridoma which can be used indefinitely to produce the antibody product either in a culture grown in the laboratory or in a live animal.

The technique has been further refined to reduce the human body's natural tendency to generate an immune response to antibodies which are produced from animal cells lines. The result is the production of *humanized* monoclonal antibodies which may be successfully administered to patients over a long period of time.

The drug Herceptin® is one of the best known success stories of this new technology. A humanized monoclonal antibody, it can bind to a protein called HER-2 which is over expressed (i.e., overproduced) on the surface of some breast cancer cells. Over-expression leads to abnormal growth signaling which leads to out-of-control cell division. Binding turns off this protein and eventually leads to cell death. Since the antibody targets only the HER-2 protein, it affects only the desired cells, thus avoiding the traditional side-effect of chemotherapy which kills all rapidly dividing cells.

Some other examples of monoclonal antibodies include Rituxan™, used to treat B-cell lymphoma; Vitaxin™, for solid tumors—now in Phase II trials; Omalizumab, for potential use in allergic asthma; Daclizumab, to prevent rejection of transplanted kidneys; and CAMPATH-1, to treat leukemia.

Avastin™, formerly known as anti-VEGF, is currently undergoing clinical trials at Genentech. The drug is another monoclonal antibody with the potential to work against solid tumors including breast cancer by binding to VEGF, a protein which acts to stimulate new blood vessel growth. It is one of a new group of emerging therapies targeted at the inhibition of such blood vessel growth, a process known as angiogenesis.

Because of their specificity and generally limited side effects, therapeutic monoclonal antibodies are under active research and development as agents to be used as adjuvant or even first-line therapies in cancer treatment. When they work, as they did for me, they can produce small miracles.

## Angiogenesis

In a series of papers during the early 1970s, Dr. Judah Folkman hypothesized and later proved that the recruitment of new blood vessels—a process known as angiogenesis—is required for tumors to grow beyond 1-2mm. He went on to develop the idea that it should be possible to starve tumors by developing therapies that would cut off their blood supply. This theory became the basis for his life-long research into the field of angiogenesis. His fascinating journey is documented in the book *Dr. Folkman's War*[12], and has

[12]    Cooke, Robert and Coop, C. Everett, *Dr. Folkman's War: Angiogenesis and the Struggle to Defeat Cancer*, Random House, 2001

spawned investigations into a number of compounds which are believed to have anti-angiogenesis potential.

Less appreciated initially, but of equally great importance, is the fact that angiogenesis is also necessary for tumor metastasis, the process by which malignant cells leave a primary tumor, enter the bloodstream, and spread to other parts of the body. Angiogenesis enhances metastasis by providing an increased density of immature blood vessels which are highly permeable to malignant cells, thus facilitating their spread into the general bloodstream. It has been estimated that as many as two million breast cancer cells can be shed into circulation each day from a 1-cm primary tumor[13], although few of these will actually develop into full-blown metastases. Animal studies have established that decreased growth of blood vessels in primary tumors is always associated with decreased formation of metastases or new tumors remote to the primary one. The converse has also been found to be true, with a strong association noted between the blood vessel density of tumors and their likelihood to metastasize in breast cancer patients.

In 1998, Dr. Folkman announced some startling laboratory results which captured intense media attention. Mice treated in his laboratory with two naturally occurring anti-angiogenesis compounds, Angiostatin and Endostatin, showed a complete regression of their tumors and were believed to be cured of cancer. This prompted his famous remark that "if you're a mouse, we can cure you of cancer." Folkman's findings have encouraged further clinical development and testing of anti-angiogenesis drugs which fall into the following general categories:

*Tumor-derived inhibitors*, a class of compounds produced naturally by tumors and which have the ability to both stimulate as well as inhibit angiogenesis. These may be produced indirectly via other tumor-generated molecules. Angiostatin and Endostatin,

---

[13]   Zetter, Bruce R., *Angiogenesis and Tumor Metastasis*, Ann. Rev. Med. 1998, 49:407-424

the first of these compounds to be identified, are believed to have a synergistic effect when combined.

Entremed, in Rockport, Maryland, is a clinical-stage biopharmaceutical company focused on the development of angiogenesis therapeutics. They have completed a number of clinical trials for Angiostatin, Endostatin and a third product candidate known as Panzem™. Current information on the status of these trials can be found at the company's website: http://www.entremed.com/pipeline.cfm

*Pharmacologic agents* have also been discovered that appear to inhibit angiogenesis. These include TNP470, an analog of the fungal antibiotic fumagillin, and Thalidomide, whose notorious effect on developing fetuses in the middle of the last century was linked to its ability to inhibit blood vessel development. In addition, several commercially available drugs used as anti-inflammatory agents are also believed to have anti-angiogenic effects. These include Celebrex® and Bextra®.

Unfortunately, the results of human trials to date have not fulfilled the promise of the earlier mouse trials. Angiostatin and Endostatin have yielded disappointing results in humans and a third drug, Avastin™, has failed to slow disease progression in a majority of breast cancer patients. Nevertheless, there have been some isolated reports that show promise including a twelve-year-old boy who was cured of a pulmonary disease resulting from excess blood vessel growth and a forty-seven-year-old woman who had her eyesight restored following treatment with Sugen 5146, an experimental anti-angiogenic pharmaceutical.

My experience with this therapy has been somewhat limited. After meeting Dr. Judah Folkman at a Stanford University seminar, I was fortunate enough to have the opportunity to solicit his advice. He recommended that I be placed on a course of treatment with Celebrex™. After consultation with my physician, I began to take this drug at a much higher level than would normally be prescribed. Unfortunately, it resulted in suppression of my blood platelets to a dangerously low level, so I had to abandon the therapy at that time. My results are inconclusive.

Despite the recent setbacks, the field of angiogenesis still appears to hold potential for the development of novel cancer treatments which could potentially be combined with others. Cancer is a complicated disease with multiple factors and pathways. I continue to watch developments in all of these fields with much interest; I would encourage you to do the same. New approaches are being developed with encouraging regularity.

## Key Insights: Emerging Therapies

- New and emerging therapies hold much promise for current as well as future cancer and breast cancer treatment.
- CyberKnife® radiotherapy is an effective and non-invasive treatment for solid tumors in the brain, spine and, to a growing extent, the lungs. Research into application to other organs is continuing.
- Radiofrequency (RF) ablation is a laparoscopic procedure for treating liver tumors, both primary and metastatic.
- Monoclonal antibody-based treatments, such as Herceptin®, have already shown success in targeting specific cancer cells which allow it to be much less toxic to the patient than traditional chemotherapies.
- The field of angiogenesis involves the discovery and development of naturally occurring, as well as man-made, pharmaceuticals in an attempt to starve tumors of their blood supply. This field continues to evolve.

# Chapter 8

## Insurance and Other Financial Issues

This section will focus on the importance, and often the difficulty, of maintaining medical, life and disability insurance in the face of ongoing illness. It concludes with some additional advice on taking care of practical matters that we all tend to ignore when healthy.

## *Medical Insurance*

Medical insurance is of paramount concern to anyone with a serious illness. Most people have no idea what is covered under their policies until they actually become sick. More frightening is the lack of knowledge about current medical costs which have the ability to break almost any budget and cause serious financial hardship, even bankruptcy. Even worse is the fact that certain types of medical care may be unavailable to those who are uninsured, under age sixty-five or make too much money to qualify for Medicaid.

While individuals and families may be able to obtain insurance on a private as well as a group basis, in general, the best coverage in this country is available through *group plans* which typically are tied to employment.

An excellent resource, "A Consumer's Guide to Getting and Keeping Health Insurance," is available online at www.healthinsuranceinfo.net. This resource covers all of the issues and much of the law associated with this issue and is searchable by state. I will highlight some of the major considerations as they pertain to the state of California, but since laws do vary by state, please refer to the online guide for the most current laws in other areas.

*Group Medical Coverage*

Group policies have several extremely important benefits for anyone who becomes ill and thereby acquires what is referred to as a "pre-existing condition." In particular, the following points are important to keep in mind:

*Some General Ground Rules:*

- Coverage under a *group* health plan *cannot be* denied or limited due to health status.
- A federal law known as HIPPA (Health Insurance Portability and Accountability Act) allows individuals to maintain coverage for pre-existing conditions when switching from one plan to another, as occurs with a change of employers, as long as there has been no more than a sixty-three-day lapse in coverage. If this period is exceeded, an applicable pre-existing condition limitation may be reduced by credits for prior coverage.
- Existing health insurance may not be cancelled due to illness.

*General Rules for COBRA Coverage*

- COBRA coverage allows an individual and/or their dependents to extend medical coverage offered by an employer when the employment relationship ends.
- All individuals with coverage from an employer who has more than fifty employees are eligible for COBRA. Premiums for COBRA coverage, identical to the employer-sponsored plan, must be paid for by the individual. The basic COBRA coverage extends insurance benefits for up to eighteen months; special circumstances—divorce, death, etc.—can extend this benefit period for up to thirty-six months.
- Individuals who are employed by employers with less than fifty employees are not protected by COBRA laws
- COBRA is available only as long as an employer offers health insurance benefits. If a company goes out of business (which

has been an issue in the high tech industry in California) or stops offering medical insurance, COBRA coverage terminates.

*Small vs. Large Group Employers*

- Small employers with two to fifty employees cannot be turned down for small group health plans, regardless of the health status of their employees. This is known as *guaranteed issuance.*
- Larger employers with more than fifty-one employees are *not* protected by guaranteed issuance. While individuals cannot be turned down for an existing plan, large groups can be turned down *as a group* due to health circumstances of individuals.

*Individual Medical Plans*

Those who are self-employed, not currently employed or whose COBRA coverage has terminated often seek to purchase medical plans on an individual basis. Some of the general, but often confusing, rules about getting private insurance include:

- Companies that sell individual health plans in California may turn down individuals who are not *federally eligible* due to their health status. This is the case even when individuals are coming directly out of group plans. It is interesting to note that this restriction varies by state. For example, New Jersey does offer guaranteed issuance for individuals previously covered by group plans.

*Federally Eligible Individuals*

- Individuals who qualify as being *federally eligible* are guaranteed the right to buy individual health plans. However, their choice of plans may be limited to two policies, either the most popular or the most representative.

- To be *federally eligible*, you must meet the following criteria:

    Eighteen months of prior creditable coverage, with the last day of coverage under a group health plan;

    You must have used up any available COBRA coverage;

    You must not be eligible for Medicare, Medicaid or a group health plan;

    You must not have health insurance;

    You must apply for coverage within the sixty-three-day window following termination of your prior policy.

- There are no pre-existing condition limitations for individuals who are federally eligible.
- Although the state limits premiums charged on policies for federally eligible individuals, they can still be quite high. However, sometimes they are the only option open to individuals who have fallen between the cracks of the health system which is largely predicated on the existence of employer-provided health insurance.

*Major Risk Medical Insurance Program (MRMIP)*

- A special risk pool program, the Major Risk Medical Insurance Program, is available through the state of California and offers health coverage for individuals who have trouble getting policies on their own. Eligibility requires one of the following:

    You must have been turned down for individual coverage (or as a member of a group of one) during the past twelve months;

Your health coverage has been involuntarily terminated during the past twelve months;

You have been offered individual coverage but at a rate that exceeds the state MRMIP rates.

*Coverage and Restrictions*:

MRMIP may stop enrolling new members for a period of time when it reaches an enrollment cap.

Coverage includes a maximum out-of-pocket amount of $2,500 for individuals and $4,000 for families, a maximum yearly benefit payment cap of $75,000 and lifetime payment cap of $750,000.

MRMIP plans have a pre-existing condition exclusion for up to six months. This can be waived if you were covered by other health insurance for at least ninety days when you applied. If you had between thirty to eighty-nine days of prior coverage, the pre-existing condition exclusion period is reduced proportionately.

If this all seems confusing, it is. However, you often have no other choice than to keep reading and asking questions until the rules become clear.

*Medicaid*

- Medicaid is a jointly-funded federal and state health insurance program for certain low-income people. It covers approximately thirty-six million individuals including children, the aged, blind and disabled, and people who are eligible to receive federally assisted income maintenance payments. Eligibility levels and benefits vary by state.

- General information on Medicaid programs can be found o

  at: http://cms.hhs.gov/medicaid

*Medicare*

- Medicare is the medical insurance plan available to all U.S. residents at age sixty-five.
- Part A offers hospital insurance and is offered without cost to anyone who has paid into the Social Security/Medicare system.
- Part B offers general medical coverage and has a monthly premium.
- In addition to those sixty-five and older, anyone who has been receiving social security disability benefits for a period of two years is automatically enrolled in both Part A and Part B in the twenty-fifth month of their disability, regardless of age.
- For detailed information, see:

  http://www.medicare.gov/

*Indigent Drug Programs*

Although the idea of facing a serious illness without any kind of health insurance is intimidating, there are some limited options for help outside the normal channels listed above. In particular, drug costs are often a very significant part of medical treatment. Many pharmaceutical companies offer what is known as an indigent drug program. Drugs covered under this program will often be made available for free or at greatly reduced cost to individuals contacting the company and asking for help. Several years ago, a friend of mine was diagnosed with breast cancer after leaving a troubled marriage, relocating to Northern California and losing her job. Although she qualified for public assistance, her benefits did not cover an expensive but particularly effective anti-nausea drug Zofran®. I contacted the company on her behalf and they sent her a simple one page application: she quickly received all the Zofran® she needed during her course of chemotherapy. This is a wonderful but little known benefit available to most anyone who asks for it and qualifies

As an example, one such program in the San Francisco Bay Area is sponsored by Genentech, the maker of Herceptin®. Their program, known as "Access to Care," can be reached at:

Genentech's Access to Care Foundation
1 DNA Way MS #13A
South San Francisco, CA 94080
(800) 530-3080.

A list of companies which offer indigent drug programs can be found at: http://www.parkinsonswellness.org/indigent.html

## Disability Coverage

Although a person in their forties is much more likely to have a long-term disability than they are likely to die, most people do not pay much attention to disability coverage until they really need it. The truth is that one in four Americans will become disabled at some point in their lives.

Disability coverage provides insurance against wages lost due to an extended illness. It typically comes in two flavors, long-term and short-term. Short-term disability typically kicks in when an illness extends past a policy-defined period of about two weeks and can run for 90 to 180 days depending on the policy. Short-term policies typically do *not* have pre-existing condition limitations which can be a huge benefit for anyone who has this issue to contend with.

Most disability policies are offered through an employer, although it is possible to obtain them on an individual basis. When paid for by an employer, the proceeds of this insurance are taxable to the individual. If the individual pays for them via payroll deduction or through a direct insurance relationship, the proceeds become tax-free, as is the case with other insurance coverage.

Salary coverage is usually limited to a maximum of 66 percent, meaning that even with this coverage in place you will still take a serious cut in pay when you cannot work. In addition, for high wage earners, there is often an eligible salary cap of $10,000 per month. Nevertheless, this is much better than the alternative of running down your savings, especially if you have an extended illness.

Many states also offer disability coverage at a much lower amount (in California, the maximum payment is $490 per week). Some employers offer this as an option to employees or as supplemental coverage. Since disability coverage is generally quite inexpensive, I would advise nearly everyone to opt for the higher paying private insurance benefit when it is available.

*Long-Term Disability*

Long-term disability coverage kicks in when the short-term policy runs out and is actually a separate policy with different rules. Probably the most important difference to note is that long-term policies almost always have *pre-existing condition limitations* which are quick to be exercised to deny payment. Unlike medical insurance, portability from one employer to another *does not exist* with respect to long-term disability and the clock begins anew with each job change.

The pre-existing condition exclusion in my policy read:

> *"Benefits will not be paid for total disability caused by, contributed to by; or resulting from; a pre-existing condition unless the Insured has been Actively at Work for one (1) full day following the end of 12 consecutive months from the date he/she became an Insured.*
>
> *Pre-existing Condition means any Sickness or Injury for which the Insured received medical treatment,*

> *consultation, care or services, including diagnostic procedures, or took prescribed drugs or medicines, during the 3 months prior to the Insured's effective date of insurance."*

Translating this into language that more of us can actually understand, it means that if you are treated for any illness or suspected illness during the ninety days before you become covered under this disability policy, the company considers that you have a pre-existing condition. You will not receive any benefits for this condition until you have been working full-time for twelve months and one day. If you must stop working full-time prior to this, the company will use the pre-existing limitation clause to deny your benefits.

Unfortunately this clause has engendered a lot of abuse by insurance companies. After my initial treatment I had decided to make a career move away from my big company job to a small startup. Four years had gone by and my doctor and I were congratulating each other on our success, believing that I might actually have been cured. Ever wary, however, I made my new employer promise to obtain disability coverage for me as a precaution; I also got a check-up and received a clean bill of health.

Just four months into the new job, I suffered a major relapse and had to take an immediate leave of absence. Since the company had purchased only long-term coverage, the ninety-day waiting period had to expire before I could make my claim.

The insurance company went through the usual process of requisitioning all of my medical records. I maintained a dialog with them which was initially friendly. Then, one day, I was informed by the claims processor that they had "found what they needed." To my surprise, coverage was denied. Although I had not had any detectable cancer cells or any treatment in the ninety days prior to the policy being put in place, I had been taking tamoxifen, which is currently being used as a preventative for both initial as well as recurrent breast cancer, for several years. Thousands of women who currently have no history of breast cancer have been enrolled in trials to see if this drug can help prevent the illness.

I filed an appeal, and my doctor wrote the following letter protesting the denial.

> *"As per our conversation earlier today the purpose of this letter is to clarify that Ms. Schreiner was on tamoxifen between 12/93 and discovery of her recurrent breast cancer in April of this year not for treatment of known disease, but rather on an adjuvant basis. Adjuvant therapy is given to patients without evidence of cancer who are considered to be at significant risk, in order to decrease the probability of recurrence. From a statistical standpoint, we know we give it to many patients who are already cured . . . Ms. Schreiner's probability of recurrence as of Jan. 1997 would have been in the range of 25% or less, given that she was then almost 4 years out with no evidence of cancer apparent."*

It was all to no avail: the conclusion was that since I had suffered a recurrence, I had never really been cured and thus, in hindsight, the tamoxifen was a treatment and not a preventative. This interpretation enabled them to apply the pre-existing condition limitation which I could not meet. This struck me as truly absurd and outrageous, but too often characteristic of the insurance industry.

With my doctor up in arms and ready to call in other medical experts, I consulted an attorney and got a quick education on ERISA, the Employee Retirement Income Security Act of 1974. This legislation covers a wide range of issues concerning employee pension plans and other benefits. Unfortunately, with respect to disability insurance, it limits recoveries to the amount that would have been paid had the policy been honored and disallows judgments for punitive damages. This creates a strong incentive for insurance companies to disallow claims based on rather flimsy arguments since they have little to lose if they unfairly deny coverage and are later found culpable.

My attorney was reluctant to handle a case which we calculated might only be worth $60,000 on a contingency basis. Since I was not in a mindset to take additional risks at that time, I reluctantly let the case drop.

To my surprise, a similar case was written up in the local newspaper about a year later, involving a woman who had also moved from a large company to a small startup. Prior to the move, she had visited her doctor for examination of a breast lump. Although she had a history of breast cancer, she had been in remission for over four years and was believed to be cured. The conclusion was that the lump was not a concern and no further action was taken at that time. She made the job change and several months later returned to her doctor for an additional exam. Unfortunately, breast cancer was diagnosed.

As a single mother of a nine-year-old and sole support of her family, disability coverage was extremely important for this woman. While she was able to collect on her short-term benefits, which typically do not have any pre-existing condition limitations, her long-term policy rejected her claim, noting that she had visited a physician within three months prior to becoming covered under the new policy and that, since she had a history of breast cancer, her condition was pre-existing. This despite the fact that the actual diagnosis was not made until much later.

The case hit the newspaper and created quite a flap, with employees offering to boycott and protest against the insurance company. Many women wrote to the newspaper citing similar examples and noted the difficulty of fighting both a serious illness and an insurance company concurrently. A few women's groups wrote their state representatives to protest the ERISA laws which fail to punish disability insurance companies for bad behavior.

Apparently the case was settled without litigation, although the settlement was never made public. All of us need to become advocates for insurance reform.

*Social Security Disability*

Individuals who have a terminal illness or who are expected to be disabled for a period in excess of a year can qualify for social security disability. The monthly benefits are based on the number of quarters of social security payments as well as the ending salary level prior to disability. Although the application process can be lengthy and cumbersome, there are services available that can act on your behalf to expedite this process. Allsup, a company located in Belleville, Illinois, provided this service for me (www.allsup.com).

Medicare coverage automatically becomes available after two years on social security disability, although coverage will not be as comprehensive as most group plans.

## Life Insurance

Life insurance is yet another tool to safeguard assets in the event of illness. The benefit to survivors is clear and needs no further explanation here. Less well-known is the fact that many life insurance policies have a living needs benefit which allows the holder to cash in up to 50 percent of benefits in advance. Life insurance can also be resold to companies who will discount the policy for cash-in-advance.

Portability and conversion are also important features of life insurance policies that anyone with a pre-existing condition should pay attention to. This allows an individual to either take an existing policy with them to a new company and/or convert a group policy to an individual basis when they leave their current employer.

## Practical Matters/Things Everyone Needs to Do

Any serious illness brings a number of issues immediately to the forefront, including financial ones. Human nature being what it is, most of us choose not to think about what will happen when we are no longer here until absolutely necessary. The truth is that everyone should pay attention to certain fundamental concerns.

## 1) Create a Will

It goes without saying that everyone should have a will prepared at some point in their lives, if only to make sure that their assets are distributed according to their wishes, as opposed to the governments'. Simple wills may be created using readily available software or with the help of a family attorney. Many people also choose to set up some type of a trust which has the benefits of avoiding probate and also some tax advantages. Estate attorneys can draft this document, often for a flat fee.

Creating a will is definitely easier to do while you are healthy and feeling well, but it's interesting to note that even for those facing more challenging situations, getting this done can create a certain sense of relief. Of more immediate concern, anyone with a serious illness needs to think about enabling others to act on their behalf in case they are temporarily disabled.

## 2) Create a Durable Power of Attorney for Health Care Decisions

Also known as an Advance Directive, this sets forth your wishes concerning medical treatment in the event you are unable to directly communicate to others. It also appoints a primary and secondary agent to act on your behalf. The form, which includes both standard options as well as space for your own specific instructions, must be signed by you and notarized. Forms are readily available from hospitals which often ask patients if they have created one.

## 3) Organize All of Your Important Documents and Records

Everyone should have some type of system to organize important documents and make them easily accessible to others in case they need to act on your behalf. I have found that binders organized by subject work well; I update them every few months. For records that are not so easy to put in binders, I use labeled file folders and/or storage boxes and filing cabinet drawers. Some key items that should be easy for others to find include:

- A list of all bank accounts, brokerage accounts, 401k plans, pension plans and any other cash or security accounts. Include copies of most recent statements in your filing system along with an asset summary sheet.
- Lists of any outstanding stock options.
- Insurance information including current policies and contacts for claims.
- A copy of your will and/or trust document.
- If you own real estate, copies of all documents related to the purchase and improvements of your properties, as well as deeds of trust.
- Tax files for the past seven years.
- Keys to safe deposit boxes.

## Key Insights: Insurance and Other Financial Concerns

- Maintaining medical insurance in the face of an ongoing disability remains a challenge in many states. In general, the most comprehensive and easiest to retain coverage is available through group plans tied to employment situations. Individuals who are unable to retain group coverage or have exhausted their COBRA coverage do have some options available to them.

  o If an individual meets the criteria for being *federally eligible*, there are some limited individual policies available. Be aware that application must be made within a narrow time window following expiration of the previous coverage.
  o Some states, such as New Jersey, do offer *guaranteed issuance* for individuals coming off of a group plan.

o The Major Risk Medical Insurance Program (MRMIP) exists as a state-managed risk pool in many states. This can offer limited coverage to individuals who cannot get it on their own.

o While Medicare covers individuals once they reach the age of sixty-five, others can also qualify if they have been receiving social security disability for two years.

o An excellent online resource for consumers covering how to get and maintain health insurance is available at: www.healthinsuranceinfo.net

• Disability plans can provide continued income during illness. Be aware that a different set of rules applies to disability coverage and claims when a pre-existing condition exists.

• Life insurance plans can sometimes be cashed in early, if needed.

• Everyone should pay attention to the creation of a will, durable power of attorney for health matters and to overall organization of their personal financial records

# Chapter 9

## The Case for Taking Charge

I have presented many examples of why taking charge of your health care can be beneficial and even life-saving. It may be easy for some to conclude that my history is an anomaly and does not actually reflect the broader state of medicine today. But I believe that a powerful argument can be made that this may be the *only* strategy in the future due to current trends in insurance, the national as well as local practice of medicine, the rapid pace of change in medical research and, perhaps most importantly, the development of an information-based society enabled by the growing resources available on the Internet.

## *Insurance Issues*

The probability of near-term passage of a comprehensive system of national healthcare insurance, single pay or otherwise, is decreasing, not increasing. At the same time, medical costs are soaring and employers and insurers are increasingly pressed to manage costs. As a result, the medical insurance industry is most likely to move from the "care for everything" model to emphasizing healthcare management and defined patient contributions. This will continue to shift the responsibility for health care management *to the individual* who will be faced with ever-increasing decisions and choices concerning their care and, ultimately, their longevity. Like it or not, individuals will eventually be brought into the system of managing their own health care dollars.

# Medical Infrastructure Issues

## Lack of a Centralized Medical Record System

Many patients have experienced the frustration of dealing with medical records, particularly if they have moved or changed physicians. Unfortunately there is no centralized system in the U.S. for documenting treatment or even managing scans such as CTs and MRIs. If there were, it might be possible for the various specialists involved to immerse themselves in the full medical picture of any given patient. Despite decades of discussion, it is unlikely—for a variety of legal, commercial, privacy and other reasons—that we will see a comprehensive system of medical records developed and deployed any time soon. This means that any long-term patient will end up managing their own records to at least some extent, often having to hand-carry them to every physician she sees. Moreover, any patient who has been through multiple courses of therapy will discover at some point that they are the *only* central repository of information about treatment they have received—something that can become critical in terms of future therapy. An example of this is a specific type of chemotherapy which involves the administration of a drug which can be cardio-toxic at certain levels. Ongoing use of this drug requires knowledge of the cumulative dose received. In order for a patient to repeat a course of treatment in the future, it is imperative for them to know the details of their prior treatments, even though that treatment may have occurred many years earlier.

## No Systematic Measurement of Quality

Likewise, there is no system of quality management in medicine: no consumer guide, no chamber of commerce, no department of consumer affairs on which one can rely to assess care. Although the AMA (American Medical Association) does exist to impose significant penalties for mistreatment (i.e., the loss of a license), there is no readily accessible public registry with which to research complaints against individual physicians. As a result, patients must rely on their own judgment, prior experience and understanding of the current standard of care when evaluating what happens to them.

## The Local Practice of Medicine

### Increasing Specialization

Driven by the pace of change, the practice of medicine continues to become increasingly specialized. Depending on the ailment, a patient may have two, three or even more physicians for various treatments. Often the patient may be the *only participant* who has all of the information and sees the full picture. I have already noted that the patient, by default, becomes the "general contractor" and must manage each of these relationships.

### Predisposition to Following a Set Course of Treatment

Many physicians have a strong emotional and personal predisposition to continue a conventional course of treatment, even when aware of alternatives which may prove to be more effective. This issue was recently addressed in a *Wall Street Journal* article, "*Too Many Patients Never Reap Benefits of Great Research*"[14], in which the author claims that "doctors often fail to pass on to patients the fruits of any discoveries." Reasons for this include the fact that some doctors take a "show-me attitude," waiting to see if treating patients according to guidelines produces better outcomes in the long run. In this situation, only an assertive and *take charge* patient can be successful in changing the treatment plan. This was evident many times when I intervened to request, and then demand, a specific treatment and switched physicians when it was denied.

---

[14]  Begley, Sharon, *Too Many Patients Never Reap Benefits of Great Research*, Wall Street Journal, Oct. 26, 2003

# The Pace of Change in Medicine

## Physician Inability to Stay Abreast of New Developments

Like many other aspects of technology, the pace of change in healthcare is so great that it is virtually impossible for clinicians, even specialists, to stay abreast of a broad spectrum of important developments relevant to any particular case. Only the patient has the motivation and, perhaps, the time to stay current.

## Easier Ways for Patients to Connect to Clinical Trials

Primarily because of the Internet, it has become much easier for patients to locate clinical trials of interest, contact researchers and enroll in trials for promising new treatments that are not yet available through their physicians. The current system of trial recruitment will continue to evolve with patients taking an active role in improving existing systems.

# Development of an Information-Based Society

Over the past several decades, the industry of information has become an integral part of our economy and, increasingly, our social structure. In the high tech industry, where I spent the majority of my professional life, information plays an especially prominent role. Thousands of market research and consulting firms spew out a mountain of reports—analyzing buyer behavior, demographic shifts, capital trends, changes in regulatory requirements and projections of what the future might hold—which are widely read by executives at all levels. There are thousands more trade show organizers—whose role is to provide a venue for companies to disseminate information about their products, which while targeted at potential customers, is also rapidly disseminated across the industry to competitors. This process ensures that all players have the information they need to survive and thrive in the market.

The same thing is true in the financial sector of our economy. When I began writing this book, the corporate financial scandals of 2002 were in full swing. At the heart of the many complaints is the allegation, apparently too often correct, that corporate executives have manipulated *information* given to investors which is needed to make intelligent investment decisions. No one has been accused of stealing money in the traditional sense; they have been accused of manipulating information for their own personal gain and to the detriment of the marketplace, underscoring the critical importance of information in our society.

Within corporations, a new set of specialists has emerged to manage and extract information so that decision makers have what they need to manage the business. Known as Information Technology (IT) or Management Information System (MIS) specialists, they have become critical to the functioning of their companies. In fact, when reduced to its most basic level, the management of *information*, the technology industry has provided much of the economic growth of a major part of the developed world for the past two decades.

In more routine transactions, every businessperson knows that being well informed is often the edge needed in any negotiation. While most patients do not consider their health care as a negotiation, there is often a subtle give-and-take in any discussion of possible treatments and cost/benefits. The well-informed patient obviously has an advantage.

At a government level, information is paramount not only to ensure management of the nation's affairs, but also for protection of its citizenry. The disastrous terrorist attacks of September 11, 2001, prompted a thorough review of the nation's intelligence gathering networks—which might have given early warning of this attack, but for many reasons failed to do so. This is perhaps the most dramatic example of the potential downside resulting from lack of information.

Information technology in medicine is generally in a backward state compared to other industries. There seems to be no medical market research available to individuals who, for a fee, could buy a report on the most effective treatments for a condition or on the most successful hospitals or the best physicians. There is little easily available public information about the efficacy of pharmaceuticals and, in fact, physicians are often bombarded by constant sales calls from competing pharmaceutical companies which have a large influence on the drugs prescribed. This is ironic because medicine clearly is a discipline where information and knowledge play important roles. Medical schools are selective institutions which accept only students who display the ability to understand and work with information about complex topics. Yet, medical informatics (the management of medical information) is an industry in its infancy by any objective measure. And where it does exist, it is aimed much more at the medical profession than at the patient.

## The Internet as the Enabling Technology

One of the most obvious trends enabling patients to play a larger role in their health care has been access to information which has exploded with the development of the Internet. Before this, it was even more difficult for patients to learn about treatment options, outcomes and everything else I have argued we all need to know to ensure high quality care. In fact, I doubt that I would have embarked on such an aggressive course without the wealth of resources available online. Many of the events in my medical life would not have been possible including access to clinical trial information (which resulted in my enrolling in a trial in Seattle), information about indigent drug programs (which enabled a friend to get free drugs during chemotherapy) and news bulletins concerning the development of Herceptin® (a drug which proved to be life-saving for me).

A recent report published by the Pew Internet and American Life Project[15], has revealed some surprising statistics about

---

[15] *Vital Decisions: How Internet users decide what information to trust when they or their loved ones are sick.* Pew Internet and American Life Project. www.pewinternet.org

Americans' use of the Internet for medical information. In a national survey conducted during March, 2002, it found that 62% of Internet users, or 73 million people (more than a quarter of the population), have gone online in search of health information. This translates into about six million people per day, or more than actually visit a health professional (office visits are estimated to be about 2.27 million per day and hospital visits, an average of 2.75 million).

In addition, almost every healthcare seeker (93 percent) has looked for information about a specific condition or illness and over half of them have gathered this information in preparation for visiting a doctor. For successful searchers, 44 percent have found online information that affected a decision about treatment and/or how to cope with a medical problem. Also reported is the fact that about one in three healthcare seekers know someone who has been helped by medical information they found online.

Physicians now routinely tell stories of patients showing up in their offices waving printouts covering the latest experimental treatments for their ailments and expecting them to be up-to-speed on everything. Interested patients can look up medical conferences relevant to their illnesses and even make arrangements to attend them if their physicians do not have the time or inclination. The most aggressive patients may be able to access new treatments to keep an illness at bay for a period of time and continue this strategy until a cure becomes available. Clearly, the Internet has made a profound difference for patients and will continue to empower them. This resource is now available to all who choose to access it and may turn out to be one of the most dramatic influences affecting the practice of medicine in this century.

All of these trends point to the increasing responsibility that patients must play in managing their own care and creating a true partnership with their physicians. The *take charge* patient will prove to be the most effective model for the future.

# Key Insights: Why You Must Take Charge

- Current trends in the practice of medicine, insurance and the pace of technological change will continue to drive increasing patient participation and responsibility.
- Near-term changes in insurance are likely to result in defined contribution accounts which will be directly managed by patients.
- The absence of a centralized medical system will drive patients to manage their own records, especially those with chronic conditions.
- The lack of any systematic quality measurement system in medicine shifts the burden of evaluation to the consumer.
- Demands on physicians' time make it increasingly difficult for them to stay abreast of the latest developments.
- Information on clinical trials will become even easier for patients to access.
- Access to a wide spectrum of information, enabled by the Internet, has empowered patients to take charge of their own health care. While this may sound like a grave responsibility to some, the truth is that active participation in determining their own treatments will prove life-saving to many. Given the current pace of medical research, even illnesses previously considered to be terminal can often be managed until the next new therapy becomes available, and, ultimately, until there is a cure.

# Chapter 10

## Living with a Chronic Illness/

## What Friends and Family Can Do

Living with a chronic, life-threatening illness is probably one of the most difficult challenges in life. You have to tap into all of your skills, problem-solving abilities and intellectual and emotional resources. Although the patient is obviously the person most directly affected, any illness also has a tremendous impact on immediate family as well as a wide circle of friends and acquaintances. In fact, it is ironic that most patients must not only muster the strength to keep themselves going but also be strong for those around them. This final chapter focuses on what friends and family can do to help as well as how my own coping strategies have evolved and changed as the journey has progressed.

### *Friends and Family Need to Deal with Their Own Feelings First*

Those nearest and dearest are often at a loss about what to do and may express feelings of helplessness. They are also torn between a desire to act as if everything will be OK and their fear that it may not. As a patient, I often felt an almost overwhelming need to protect them from bad news. Although I firmly believe that maintaining a positive attitude is enormously helpful, it can occasionally feel like an additional burden.

People close to the patient must first come to terms with their own feelings. The initial challenge is conquering their own fear of the illness as well as thoughts of their own mortality. I think this is particularly difficult if the patient is relatively young. Although there may be a time when it is appropriate to discuss end-of-life issues, most patients do not actively think about dying; they are focused on survival and quality of life. Learning more about the course of an illness and its treatments can often help to demystify the situation and make it more approachable.

## Realize that Chronic Illness Is Different from Acute Illness

Although both chronic and acute illnesses are challenging, I believe that chronic illness is actually more difficult. Acute situations tend to arouse instant sympathy as people rally to support the patient. The situation, although often frantic, is usually resolved fairly quickly. Life returns to normal in a fairly short time and everyone resumes their usual routines. Chronic illnesses, however, involve a prolonged battle with many ups and downs and the inevitable changes and adjustments in daily life. Despite a lot of support from others, I often felt quite removed from what I considered to be a normal life with its structure and daily consideration of issues both large and small. It was—and continues to be—a lonely and isolating experience that only others facing a similar set of constraints can truly appreciate. For patients and those close to them, life is often changed permanently.

## Practical Things

How can friends and family help? In practical terms, they can give freely of their time and attention to the extent they are able. Since patients dealing with an ongoing situation are often loath to ask for help, others should be aware that it is important for them to take the initiative. Meal preparation, visits to the hospital and offers of rides to doctors' appointments will be appreciated even if they are not actively solicited or even necessary. Accompanying a patient to a difficult session can be useful even if it does no more than offer a physical presence. Beyond that, it is good to have another set of eyes and ears along, someone to take notes that can be reviewed following a consultation, particularly when important decisions must be made. This frees the patient to focus on what the physician is saying as opposed to transcribing every detail.

People who really want to help in a significant way can get busy reading the chapters covering outside research, educating themselves and becoming involved in the search for alternative therapies, including clinical trials. This takes a major commitment in terms of time and focus which will be greatly appreciated. I was fortunate to have had one friend, Joanne (a fellow breast cancer survivor), who actually did more research on emerging therapies than I did. Her constant search for new information was both practical as well as a source of enormously positive support. I felt that she was always looking out for my future.

People who are limited in their ability to provide direct help, or are still struggling with their own feelings of discomfort, can do something simple like sending a card or a note that lets the patient know they are thinking of them.

## *Realize It's a Different Reality*

Friends and family should also realize that the "world of the sick" is quite different from the everyday world they experience. It is full of hospitals, doctors, nurses, blood transfusions, chemotherapy and its own infrastructure that operates in quite a different mode than their daily experience. This compounds the feelings of being different and the isolation that many patients experience.

On a day-to-day level, it can be helpful to bring the outside world to the patient during periods of extended hospitalization and/or convalescence. I have a distinct memory of one colleague,

Marian, who called me a number of times during my stem cell transplant and gave me reports on the politics going on in Italy where she was temporarily assigned. I don't know if she realized how good it was for me to be, at least temporarily, drawn back into the real world.

## Don't Treat the Patient Differently

The majority of patients do not want to be treated as if they are cancer patients. While some do succumb to the notion of being sick, a surprising number do not want to be defined by their illness and make every effort to deal with it as just another one of life's challenges. Unless circumstances dictate otherwise, friends and family should maintain the same expectations for the patient that they have always had. Encourage them to maintain an active life.

## Don't Ask the Patient How She Got the Disease

Many breast cancer patients are surprised by the fact that they are approached repeatedly by friends and colleagues who want to know how they contracted breast cancer. The underlying message is that they want to know so that they can avoid that behavior and reduce their own risk.

The fact is that the majority of breast cancer patients have no known risk factors. The causes remain relatively little known beyond risks conferred by genetically inherited mutations, which represent only a small percentage of cases. Most cancer patients have done nothing wrong and do not appreciate being made to feel that the illness is somehow their fault. Be sensitive to this issue.

## Don't Panic

Supporters should also try to avoid over-reacting, particularly when new challenges arise. Since panic is contagious, this often just adds to the patient's stress. Nor should others ignore a serious situation or attempt to make light of it. The appropriate response is often a difficult balance of concern mixed with a resolve to get past the current situation.

## Be There and Don't Give Up

Almost all patients harbor the fear that they will be abandoned when the going gets rough. This is not always rational: it usually stems from the concern that the experience will be so negative that others will get tired of dealing with it, give up and go away. Unfortunately, this may be reinforced by the behavior of some friends who *do* shy away at the time of the initial diagnosis. It is extremely important to communicate—in whatever way appropriate—that you'll be there for the long haul. *No matter what.*

## Enjoy the Good Times

Although cancer is certainly a challenge, it's not necessarily a death sentence. Even when it does have a sad outcome, many patients live quality lives for many years. It is important to realize that there will be many positive times when the illness is either in remission or has only a minor impact. Enjoy them and resume life on a normal basis.

## Personal Coping Strategies

Some of my own personal coping mechanisms have already been mentioned where I reflect on the many challenges that breast cancer has presented. My major strategy has been to maintain an active lifestyle and focus on activities which absorb me and provide a distraction from the medical problems. This has been easiest when I have been working, even on a part-time basis.

During this latest bout, I decided to temporarily withdraw from work because of all of the logistical problems associated with being a cancer patient as well as the uncertainty involved in dealing with metastatic illness. This has been particularly difficult and has required a lot of adjustment on many levels. With the pinnacle of my career in sight, it was tough to back away from long-held career aspirations. A return to work was one of my early coping strategies which always had the effect of satisfying my need for accomplishment, returning my life to some semblance of normality and preventing me from dwelling too much on the downside.

The issue of work deserves a bit more attention, since it is so problematic for many. Of particular importance is the concern that many patients have of telling others about their struggles. This is a tricky subject, since people dealing with serious illness can suffer from subtle discrimination in jobs they already hold and may also encounter difficulty in searching for new jobs. I must admit that during the course of my treatments, I employed different tactics at different times depending on the situation. When I was initially diagnosed, I had been employed by a large computer company, established a good reputation and had little concern about job security. I was quite open about my diagnosis and, in fact, often wore a scarf to work during chemotherapy when I tired of the wig. I don't believe that my illness was a significant factor with respect to my tenure there.

However, many years later, I joined a startup in the midst of the mania that swept Silicon Valley during the go-go dot-com years. It was a high stress, highly competitive period; I knew that my medical history would, at best, be viewed neutrally and, at worst, as a negative. Since I was enjoying a remission at that time, I decided to keep quiet about my past. I believe it was the correct decision.

I have seen patients on both ends of the spectrum, those who have been remarkably open about their situations as well as those who have told almost no one, including their closest friends. The downside of withholding is, of course, that you get no support from others. The upside is that you may be spared some level of discrimination which will be difficult to detect. This is a very personal decision.

The early battle was characterized much more by crisis, by learning and the constant search for new information. The current struggle is characterized more by the acceptance of an ongoing, difficult situation that dominates and has totally changed my life. Despite this, I consider most days to be pleasant and have learned to deal resolutely with the challenges. Life has now taken on a slower pace, consisting of a variety of personal projects including the writing of this book, a major landscaping remodel and the week-to-week logistics of dealing with a chronic illness.

Probably the most frustrating thing at this point is the difficulty in making both long-term and sometimes even short-term plans. With no remission in sight, and tied to a weekly treatment regimen which may become complicated by additional therapy needed to counteract side effects, it is difficult to travel very far or make extended commitments. In this sense, the usual benefits of "retirement" have been elusive. Nevertheless, I remain mostly positive and celebrate the small victories. I continue to look forward to a time when I can resume work, which is not entirely out of the question at this point. And Dave and I still continue to *plan for the future*. In fact, we have just planted a small vineyard which will not bear fruit for several years. I have every intention of being there for the first harvest.

I am often asked by friends how I manage to deal with the situation in such a matter-of-fact way. The truth is that I have always resisted letting the illness define who I am. Even after ten years of therapy, I often walk into a treatment room thinking that I don't really belong there. In fact, since I have continued to "look good," other patients often look puzzled by my presence. I attribute a large part of this to my adherence to a daily exercise regimen which includes weight-lifting and jogging on a treadmill. Although every setback has made the resumption of exercise more difficult, I do believe that it is the key to a long and healthier life. I was recently pleased to discover that a friend on the East Coast thought I was actually five years younger than I am. This was truly a remarkable compliment, considering all the therapy I've had!

Although cancer is a large part of my life, I take every opportunity to relegate it to a lesser priority and deal with it as just one of many activities. This seems to have the effect of making the entire process less threatening for others, who then find it easier to offer support. Since support is so important to anyone with a critical illness, this actually has become not only an effective coping strategy but also a survival strategy since others are drawn closer.

Almost anyone with a serious illness will tell you that it has been a life-altering event. Ironically, it takes something that threatens us immediately in order to force us to realize that life is short. Following the events of 9/11, I often felt that the entire country had suffered a near-death experience and was reacting in a similar way to patients who have been given a dire prognosis. The stages are much the same: shock, denial, anger and, finally, acceptance of what has happened and the ability to live with it.

Although my determination to keep battling continues unabated, I live much more in the moment with a deeper sense of appreciation and consciousness of limits. My family and friends are of primary importance to me. I also consider it a priority to do what I can to help others in similar situations, which is the primary motivation for this book. From discussions with others, I believe this to be a universal reaction to the experience.

I have worked hard to retain my sense of humor which has always gotten me through difficult situations. I often quote one of my physicians who, noting that I had survived my stem cell transplant, playfully commented that I was "hard to kill." I intend to stay that way!

I continue to be amazed at the capability of people to get through the most challenging of circumstances. Although many people have told me that they could never have handled such a difficult situation, I believe that you never know until you are tested. Most of us are more resilient than we think. In the end, the most important thing is not to give up hope.

I'm still here, still fighting, ever hopeful.

# Appendix

## Summary of Online Resources

### Patient Educational Services:

| | |
|---|---|
| Planetree Health Resources Centers | www.planetree.org |
| Community Breast Health Project | www.cbhp.org |
| Bay Area Breast Cancer Network | www.babcn.org |

### Top Ten Most Useful Health Sites*

| | |
|---|---|
| Centers for Disease Control | www.cdc.gov |
| Healthfinder | www.healthfinder.gov |
| HealthWeb | www.healthweb.org |
| HIV InSite | www.hivinsite.ucsf.edu |
| Mayo Clinic | www.mayoclinic.com |
| Medem | www.medem.com |
| MEDLINEplus | www.medlineplus.gov |
| National Women's Health Info Center | www.4women.gov |
| NOAH (NY Onlince Access to Health) | www.noah-health.org |
| Oncolink | ww.oncolink.upenn.edu |

### Clinical Trials

| | |
|---|---|
| PDQ/National Cancer Institute | www.cancer.gov |
| National Library of Medicine/NIH | www.clinicaltrials.gov |
| CenterWatch | www.centerwatch.com |
| Emerging Med | www.emergingmed.com |

## Sources for Medical News:

| | |
|---|---|
| PR News Wire | www.prnewswire.com/news/ |
| EurekaAlert! | www.eurekalert.org |
| Biospace | www.biospace.com/news |
| Business Wire (use search) | www.businesswire.com |
| Breast Cancer News | www.breastcancer.net |

## Specialized Patient Services:

| | |
|---|---|
| CAN (Corporate Angels Network) | www.corpangelsnetwork.org |

## Medical Conference Information:

| | |
|---|---|
| Medscape | www.medscape.com |

## Medical Research:

| | |
|---|---|
| National Library of Medicine | www.nlm.nih.gov/ |
| Medline/Pub Med | www.ncbi.nlm.gov/ entrez/query.fcgi |

## Emerging Therapies:

| | |
|---|---|
| Accuray Inc (Cyberknife) | www.accuray.com |
| Rita Medical Systems | www.ritamedical.com |
| Radiofrequency Ablation | http://rfa.ucsf.edu |
| Entremed | www.entremed.com |

## Insurance/Financial Issues:

| | |
|---|---|
| Consumers' Guide to Insurance | www.healthinsuranceinfo.net |
| Medicaid | http://cms.hhs.gov/medicaid |
| Medicare | www.medicare.gov/ |

Allsup                              www.allsup.com
Indigent Drug Programs              w w w . p a r k i n s o n s
                                    w e l l n e s s . o r g /
                                    indigent.html

\*      according to the Pew Internet and American Life Project

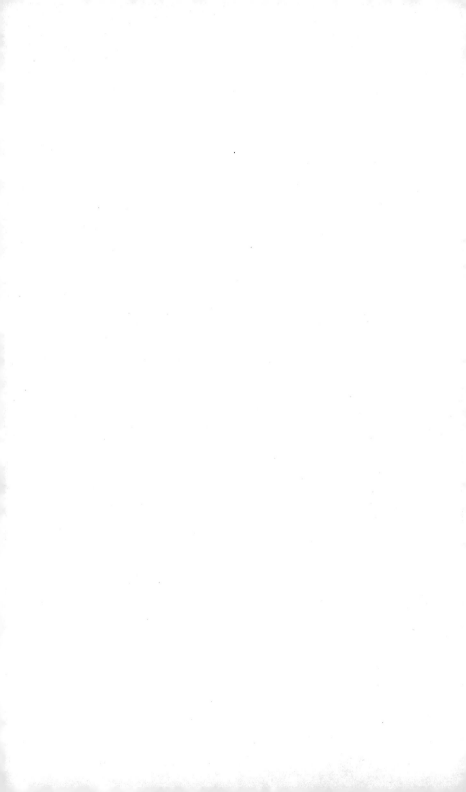

# Index

# R

# S

# T

# V

# Z

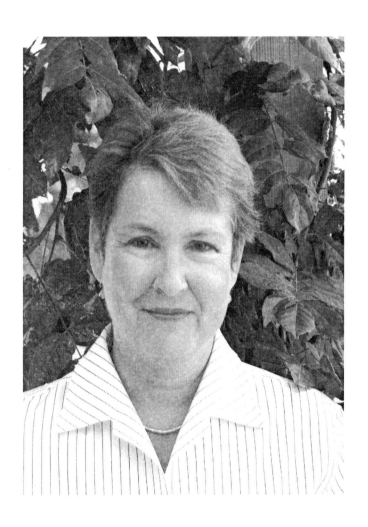

# About the Author

Joan Schreiner has successfully battled breast cancer for more than ten years. During the course of this struggle, she has become active in numerous breast cancer groups, been a speaker at medical conferences, a participant in a clinical trial, an author of articles for local breast cancer newsletters, and featured on both radio and in a television documentary about surviving breast cancer.

A graduate of U.C. Berkeley with a B.S. in Nutrition Science, Joan worked as a chemist at Stanford University for two years before returning to her alma mater to earn an MBA in Finance. During her 20-year career, she held increasingly responsible positions in corporate finance for such well-known Silicon Valley companies as Intel, Convergent Technologies, and Silicon Graphics. In 1997, she left big company life to join and advise a series of start-ups, winding up as VP Finance/CFO for Shutterfly, an online photofinisher, which allowed her to combine business with her passion for photography.

Due to her continuing struggle with breast cancer, Joan retired from full-time work in 2001 to focus on writing this book and launching an internet-based registry for breast cancer patients who want to be matched to clinical trials, a project hosted by the Carol Franc Buck Breast Care Center at the University of California, San Francisco.

Joan lives in Los Gatos with her husband, David Nagel, and Webster, their beloved golden retriever. Together, they have planted a small vineyard in the Santa Cruz Mountains. She intends to be there for the first harvest.

Joan can be reached with questions and/or comments at:

*joanschreiner@att.net*